Woman of few Words

*My Creative Journey
with Dystonia*

Cheri Tannenbaum

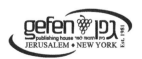

gefen נפן
publishing house בית הוצאת לאור
JERUSALEM ♦ NEW YORK   Est. 1981

Cover Design: Dragan Bilic
Typeset in Arno Pro by Raphaël Freeman, Renana Typesetting

ISBN: 978-965-229-973-4

1 3 5 7 9 8 6 4 2

Gefen Publishing House Ltd.   Gefen Books
6 Hatzvi Street   140 Fieldcrest Ave.
Jerusalem 94386, Israel   Edison NJ, 07081
+972-2-538-0247   516-593-1234

orders@gefenpublishing.com
www.gefenpublishing.com

Grateful permission is acknowledged for permission to reproduce
quotes from Rabbi David Aaron, Dr. Miriam Adahan, Aish.com,
Maureen Bogoroch-Ditkofsky, Chabad.org, Daily Emunah, Rebbetzin Tziporah
Heller, John J. Heney, Brenda Currey Lewis, Mishpacha magazine, Moe Mernick,
Rabbi Dovid Orlofsky, Orit Esther Riter, Rebbetzin Shira Smiles, Rabbi Yechiel Spero,
Rabbi Baruch Taub, Toras Avigdor, and Rabbi Dr. Abraham J. Twerski.

Printed in Israel

* * *

Library of Congress Cataloging-in-Publication Data

Names: Tannenbaum, Cheri, 1952- author.
Title: Woman of few words : My creative journey with dystonia / Cheri Tannenbaum.
Description: Jerusalem : Gefen Publishing House Ltd. ; Edison, NJ : Gefen
  Books, [2019]
Identifiers: LCCN 2019017482
Subjects: LCSH: Tannenbaum, Cheri, 1952- | People with
  disabilities--Biography. | Dystonia musculorum deformans--Popular works. |
  People with disabilities--Religious aspects--Judaism.

Contents

Foreword by Rav Avi Weiss   ix

Preface   xi

Acknowledgments   xiii

Prologue   xv

1   My Early Life   1

2   Young Adulthood   8

3   The Epitome of Health   18

4   Building Our Family   24

5   Challenges and Opportunities   44

6   Milestones   56

7   Let My Right Hand Forget Its Skill   67

8   Moments of Joy   73

9   Thoughts on Living Without   77

10   What I Have Learned   101

Appendix I: Letters from Family and Friends   112

Appendix II: What Is Dystonia?   122

Appendix III: Inspirational Quotes   127

To my husband Harvey and our three children,
Orit, Nechama and Simcha

And to my mother, may she live and be well,
and my father, of blessed memory

Foreword by Rav Avi Weiss

There is a tradition that names, even names that are not Jewish, when written out phonetically in Hebrew, have inner meaning. This teaching is especially appropriate for Cheri.

In Hebrew, Cheri is *shiri* – literally, my song. In the Torah, God tells us to write *hashirah hazot* (this song), referring, according to most commentators, to the whole of the Torah itself. From this perspective, the Torah is not only a holy work to be studied, but a song, a melody, a sweetness that encompasses the history, the aspirations, a guide to living for all of Am Yisrael.

Over the years I've read many works which try to describe the Torah's melodious teachings. But for me, the best book one can read is to observe the way Cheri lives. Cheri, on every level, lives and breathes the words of the Torah – she walks with God.

Rav Kook once wrote that every soul is a song. There are those who sing the song of their inner selves; and then there are those whose song extends beyond themselves – to their family. And then there are souls that are so deep and so high they embrace all of Am Yisrael, even the world. This is Cheri's songful soul.

I'm delighted that Cheri has finished this extraordinary volume, as every time I see Cheri, every time I have the honor to speak with her, I feel uplifted. I feel I'm in the presence of greatness. I feel and can hear the song that is sung by the angels themselves. I have little doubt that anyone who reads Cheri's book will be similarly uplifted.

Dear Cheri, for me, you have always been a profile in courage. From the time you were a student thirsting for knowledge of Torah, to the difficult moments when facing a serious physical challenge, to the glorious moment when you married Harvey and then, against all odds, with God at your side, brought children into the world – you have been a song that stands above and apart from all others.

Cheri, as you reach this wonderful milestone, Toby joins me in offering our blessings to you for health, life, and fulfillment. May you continue being an inspiration, fulfilling the words of Solomon the King, who wrote that there are those who rise above all others, impacting their family, Am Yisrael, and the world.

With gratitude, respect, and endless friendship,

RAV AVI

Preface

How would you like to be unable to speak intelligibly? How would you enjoy having an awkward gait that makes you prone to falling and causes people to stare as you shuffle by? Living with dystonia is not something I would have chosen for myself. To tell the truth, what I really long for is normalcy. Better yet, I'd like to go away somewhere and not take myself with me! Wherever I go, people are always telling me that I am an inspiration. This makes me feel like a total fraud, because to my mind I'm just doing what I have to do to drag myself out of bed every morning and face another day of humiliation and challenges.

But then again, I could have made the choice to just stay in bed and pull the covers over my head and never get up, so I suppose the fact that I do get up day after day could be seen as a source of inspiration. Honestly, being put on an "inspiration pedestal" can be somewhat isolating. (Think about it: Would you rather have people gush that they're in awe of you or just be the friend people want to hang out with?)

But if others see me as an inspiration, I consider it an honor. And if my struggles can help others, then my suffering has purpose and ennobles me.

This is why I have taken the opportunity to write a book sharing my philosophy on how to be a functioning human being despite stark challenges, and how to leave your mark on this world.

I do hope that this book serves as an inspiration to all those who have been tested by God through a disability. I fervently believe that, with faith, courage, and fortitude, you can live a fulfilling life, one full of happiness, blessings, and contentment.

This is how it can be done.

Cheri Tannenbaum
July 2019
cherbelz@yahoo.com

Acknowledgments

My deepest thanks to my dear family: Harvey, Orit, Nechama, and Simcha, as well as my sons-in-law and grandchildren.

Harvey, how can I thank you enough for your support all these years?

I know it was not easy for any of you, my children, to be raised by a mother who is different because of a disability. Nonetheless, it has undoubtedly strengthened all of you, and I am happy to see that you seem to have suffered no harm from it.

On the contrary, I think this has been a deeply character-building experience, which has taught you empathy, sympathy, and kindness. It has given you the strength of your convictions and has taught you how to give to others. These are all important attributes that will serve you well in life.

You have all served as my voice and legs, which has added meaning and depth to all our lives. I am deeply grateful to you for always worrying about, keeping an eye on, and taking such good care of me.

A part of me always feels bad that it shouldn't be the job of young children to take care of their mother; it should be the mother who takes care of her children. However, my cousin Eric told me I should be grateful that my children are sensitive enough to recognize and meet my special needs. And, indeed, I truly am. I thank them profusely and apologize for the situation. In some ways, my affliction probably forced them to grow up too fast.

I would also like to thank my mother and father, to whom I owe a lot of *hakarat hatov* (gratitude) for giving birth to me, raising me, and for starting the Dystonia Medical Research Foundation in the hopes of finding a cure for me. I knew I could count on them to be there for me at any time of the day or night, in good times and in bad. I also thank them for cheering me on to finish my book, knowing how important it is to others with disabilities.

Sadly, my father died in March 2018, before the publication of this book. He was a successful, self-made businessman who also became well known for his philanthropy. This included providing the seed money for the establishment of the Simon Wiesenthal Center in Los Angeles, cofounding the Yeshiva University High School in Los Angeles, establishing Action Canada (a nonprofit leadership development initiative), and founding the Dystonia Medical Research Foundation. May his memory be for a blessing.

I'd like to thank Gefen Publishing House – including Publisher Ilan Greenfield, Project Managers Devorah Beasley and Daphne Abrahams, and Senior Editor Kezia Raffel Pride – for bringing my dream to fruition.

I would also like to thank Steve Ganot and Jill Rogoff for their assistance with my manuscript in its earlier stages.

Finally, I'd like to thank Hakodosh Baruch Hu for giving me this test to enable me to help others get through theirs.

Prologue

One night, I was in the kitchen with my mother, helping her prepare a salad. When she spoke to me, I suddenly found myself unable to answer.

Since 1972, I have suffered from a neurological movement disorder called dystonia musculorum deformans. Dystonia is not my essence, nor does it define me. It is the mark of an enigma that I wear with pride.

Nonetheless, because – unfortunately – it has played a key role in my life, my story cannot be understood without knowing something about dystonia. According to the Dystonia Medical Research Foundation, this disorder affects some 300,000 people in North America alone. Its causes are unknown, as yet, but research has found that those who consistently make high-precision hand movements (e.g., engineers, artists, architects, and musicians) are particularly vulnerable. It comes in many forms, some of which affect only localized parts of the body; other forms, however, affect larger areas, and those suffering from it often make repetitive twisted movements and assume awkward positions. Some forms of dystonia appear in early childhood, and some (like mine) are late onset.

The specific type of dystonia that I have remains unknown to date. What I do know is that I will be bearing it for as long as God deems that I should. But for how long? Forever?

If you break your little finger, you may only be reminded of the pain when you need to use that body part. Dystonia is not like that: it is my constant companion, accompanying my every step and every breath. I wake up to it each morning and go to sleep with it each night.

I never asked for this affliction and would willingly forgo its company; but it is here, inhabiting my entire body. Anytime I need to make a move, there it is. And anytime I want to speak, there it is again. For just one second, I would like a reprieve. I long for one second of "normalcy," but it is not to be: I am meant to be burdened with it, unless someday my wish is fulfilled.

In my finiteness, I am totally enraged at what I feel to be the unfairness of my affliction. In His infiniteness, God feels that – for some reason that only He is privy to – I need this test for myself and for the world. The foundational Jewish theologian Rav Moshe Chaim Luzzatto in his classic work *Derech Hashem* (The Way of God) explains that tests from God are an opportunity to actualize our potential, to find out what we are made of. It is only by being tested that we discover our unique mission in life.

I was moved by the words of Jewish writer Chana Kroll, who wrote, "When confronted with pain, we have three choices. We can pretend it isn't there and think about something else – simple escapism. We can dwell on it without doing anything about it – though that can lead to depression. Or we can recognize it is a sign that something isn't what it's supposed to be – and seek to fix it."[1]

Since the dystonia first presented, I have gone back and forth repeatedly between all three of these states. I can try to fix it, giving it my all; however, I must not forget that the outcome is totally in God's hands.

I do not know whether I could have coped with and found

---

1. Chana Kroll, "Bitterness Moves: Parshat Beshalach," TheJewishWoman.org, https://www.chabad.org/theJewishWoman/article_cdo/aid/470961/jewish /Bitterness-Moves.htm. Used by permission of Chabad.org.

meaning in my condition without developing a personal philosophy that carries me – day by day – from one challenge to the next. The philosophy I try to live by is that we are here on earth to overcome the challenges and to allow ourselves to be filled with joy. Of course, I did not make it up myself, but rather combined the lessons I have gleaned from a variety of sources and applied them to my life in a way that makes sense to me. Others may develop somewhat different approaches that better help them deal with their own unique challenges. I hope, however, that they may benefit from whatever wisdom and experience I have gained over the years, just as I have learned from others.

From Chabad Rebbetzin Chana Weisberg, editor of TheJewishWoman.org, I learned that, while battling adversity – whether a physical affliction like mine or any other significant challenge – three important tenets should be kept in mind:

1. Your battles don't define you. Even if your battles are constant, you are not your battles. You will win some and lose some, but the triumphs cannot improve, nor can the losses damage, your divine soul, which is already perfect.
2. You are not fighting alone. God is on your side and will provide the help you need, in His own way, in His own time.
3. You can grow from your experience. Whatever challenge you have, it is for a good reason, and can be harnessed for self-improvement.[2]

Remaining faithful to these fundamentals can be difficult when facing such a test from God. Every challenge, large or small (and

---

2. Adapted from Chana Weisberg, "Who Are You Fighting Today? 3 Steps to Victory," TheJewishWoman.org, August 23, 2015, https://www.chabad.org/blogs/blog_cdo/aid/3025116/jewish/Who-Are-You-Fighting-Today.htm. Used by permission of Chabad.org.

everyone thinks his or her personal challenge is a large one), is a test that He has specifically designed for that individual.

Rabbi Avigdor Miller says of the necessity of such tests:

> We have to be tested, otherwise you can ask why do you need this world at all; we should all be in Gan Eden [the Garden of Eden], together with the Shechina [the presence of God]. We see this is a world where difficulties are erected as barriers, as hurdles for us and that's our success: despite the difficulties, to succeed in making out of ourselves the best that we can.[3]

We are here on earth to overcome the challenges and to allow ourselves to be filled with joy – hence my continual smile.

Each test that a person faces is tailor made by the Almighty for that specific individual, to give him the tools that he needs to grow and uncover his hidden spiritual, emotional, mental, and physical potential. Self-examination is the ultimate challenge. It includes making every effort not to succumb to the "grass is always greener" syndrome by comparing our lives with those of others.

We can never measure the pain of others, nor stand in their shoes. Consequently, none of us can objectively determine whether our pain is more or less severe than that of someone else. People say to me, "I feel so bad telling you my worries; yours are so much worse." Please do not ever be embarrassed to complain to me. You are mistaken; your pain is as pervasive to you as mine is to me. We are together in our suffering, as each person is as overwhelmed by his troubles or pain as the next. It can be helpful to commiserate with others and learn different coping skills from each other. No one said

---

3. Rabbi Avigdor Miller, *SimchaMinute* by Rabbi Avigdor Miller, "Waiting for Moshiach," no. 795, cited on Living with Hashem, December 30, 2015, http://www.livingwithhashem.com/lwh-blog-posts/make-something-out-of-yourself. Used by permission of Toras Avigdor.

life would be easy, but it can be filled with happiness and meaning if we learn how to embrace all that it brings to us.

As Moe Mernick wrote, "Only once you embrace what you have been given – yes, that means every aspect of that package – can you truly lead a happy life. We should not feel that we are being held back by our challenges, instead they should propel us forward."[4]

Hopefully, you can face your own problems in your own way and in your own time and arrive at a far more appropriate and helpful response than "Why me?"

> Don't say why is this happening to me – rather say now that this is happening to me, what is this happening asking of me. Let the happening ask what can I learn from this. How can I become a better person, a more focused person, etc. This will set my mind and soul to look for an answer... [5]

How much more meaningful it is to ask, *What does God want from me? How can I use this as a vehicle to bring out my hidden potential? How can this bring me closer to God? How can I use this difficulty to help make an impact on the world, to bring good into the world and to be a shining light to all the other nations?*

When used in this way, pain is a potent spiritual tool: God sends us challenges to help us access deeper levels of spiritual intention and passion. When we use our troubles as a tool to come closer to God, we transform difficulties into spiritual elevations.

But what do you do with your anger? If you do not have any, more power to you!

We are told that God suffers with us in our pain, and that He has given us this test and can take it away whenever He wants to. I have

---

4. Moe Mernick, *The Gift of Stuttering: Confronting Life's Challenges; A Personal Journey* (Bet Shemesh: Mosaica Press, 2016), 85. Used by permission of Moe Mernick.
5. Rabbi David Aaron. Used by permission of Rabbi David Aaron.

heard it said that pain should not be interpreted as a punishment, but rather as a corrective, given to us by a loving God Who wants only our good. If we only understood the benefit we get from our trials, goes the maxim, we would ask for this pain to be given to us!

How does this affect our relationship with God? Our sages say that everything that happens to you – every *nisayon* (test) that comes your way – is exactly what you need for your spiritual growth. It is exactly what you need to grow and become closer to Hashem (God). In my case I didn't feel that at all. I was stagnating. I couldn't move, literally and figuratively. I was in constant survival mode, with no life force spurring me on. I was totally self-absorbed.

Ideally, recognizing that only God has the choice of whether and how to help us should draw us closer to Him, as He is our sole source of salvation. However, what if, instead, such recognition of God's power over us turns us away from Him, alienating us, causing us to feel unloved by Him and resentful that we have been picked on for some unknown reason?

You could look at it another way. The word *nisayon* [test] has the word *nes* in it, which means miracle: "The test is there to bring out the miracle in you. To elicit strength that is uncharacteristic and unfamiliar."[6] God is not picking on you. Rather, "He's training you to be miraculous."[7]

It is difficult to internalize, but it's important to realize that our pain is given to us out of deep love.

We must never think that because we have questions, God doesn't love us every bit as much. He knows that we sometimes struggle. But He always brings us close, gives us a kiss on our

---

6. Rochel Holzkenner, "Faith under Fire," Chabad.org, https://www.chabad .org/parshah/article_cdo/aid/2739619/jewish/Faith-Under-Fire.htm. Used by permission of Chabad.org.

7. Ibid.

forehead, and lets us know that in spite of all our questions, He loves us more than anything.[8]

Suffering is not meant to crush us but rather to expand us.

> When a person is suffering, he may feel that all doors are closed to him. He cannot live the life he envisioned for himself or achieve what he had hoped to accomplish. In actuality when Hashem punches us down His purpose is to open new doors for us enabling latent qualities to emerge so that we can refine ourselves.[9]

I always wear an upbeat look on my face, hoping it will be infectious and that people will see the real me and not my disability. No one wants to be confronted by an unhappy expression. My bright and cheery face serves to uplift my own spirits and keeps me from bringing pain into the lives of all the people that I meet.

I've also acquired the habit of dressing to the nines to make myself look and feel interesting and to help me personify God's glory. In this way, I feel more empowered and presentable while always helping to serve a greater purpose.

A disability is only limiting if you allow it to take over and define who you are as a person. I feel an obligation to share my story to help inspire others who are also struggling with disabilities. It is entirely possible to live a productive life and contribute to your family and community while living with a disability. Director of the Jewish National Fund's Task Force on Disabilities Yossi Kahana points out that Moses himself had a speech impediment, yet didn't let this stop him from becoming the paradigmatic Jewish leader: "These are the facts; we have everything to give – if society can learn

---

8. Rabbi Yechiel Spero, *Inspiration Daily*, Yeshiva Ateres Shimon. Used by permission of Rabbi Yechiel Spero.
9. Rebbetzin Suri Gibber. Used by permission of *Mishpacha* magazine.

to move past nature's constraints and facilitate our abilities."[10] The fact that I have a disability doesn't mean that I don't have anything to give. I need the world to look beyond my disability and help me show my abilities.

A woman who suffered paralysis after a mismanaged epidural put it this way: "I *have* a disability and I also *have* illnesses, but I am NOT the disability, nor am I the illness. I am a woman, healthy in my mind, in my attitude, in my approach to life. And if I can't get out of bed today because of pain or other issues, well thank God tomorrow is another day!"[11]

Every religious philosopher must grapple with a basic quandary: Why does God, Who is all-knowing, all-powerful, and all-good, allow suffering? Attempts to answer this are called theodicies, and many have been offered – some more satisfying and convincing than others. I am not aware of any theodicies that solve the question forever, but one that has made a lot of sense to me was expressed in homiletic form by Shmuel Pollen on the Chabad.org website. Here is an excerpt.

> You are playing a game called "My Perfect Life." Every day, you strive to have perfect health, perfect finances and the perfect marriage. Or as close as you can get to them. When suffering occurs, you're angry because that means your game is being ruined.
>
> What game is G-d playing? It's called "The Perfect *Story*." G-d wants to tell the greatest story ever told....
>
> So where are you in this game? You're on camera! You're an actor and He's the Director. You've been in this movie the whole

---

10. Yossi Kahana, "D'var Torah for Jewish Disabilities, Awareness, Acceptance, and Inclusion Month," https://www.jnf.org/menu-2/ways-to-help/jewish-disabilites-awareness-acceptance-and-inclusion-month.

11. Michele Thaler, "I Am Not My Disability," Aish.com, Jun 10, 2017, https://www.aish.com/ci/s/I-Am-Not-My-Disability.html. Used by permission of Aish.com.

time. The problem is, you don't realize you're in it.... Until one day, you decide to listen. The words you hear affect you to the very core of your being. You begin to feel like you've awakened from a bad dream.... Things begin to come into focus...

This is what the Director said: "My child, I chose you for this specific role for a reason. I waited a long time for you to turn to Me and find out what it was.... Your role is to find a way to be a hero for someone else....

"I wish you would uplift others who have fallen, with a kind word or a small act of charity. I wish you would feel grateful for all of the good that surrounds you, and that you would humbly accept the challenge to overcome the rest....

"And where will I be?.... I will be with you in that moment of pain... Because we are not separate.... And you will never be alone....

The challenges will be there. They aren't torture. They are the Director's way of saying, "I believe in you. I have a lesson that I need to teach the audience, and I think you can do it like no one else in the world...."

You can never lose. Because the failures are worth just as many points as the successes....

The Director's instructions are the Torah and its mitzvahs.... The day is coming when only good things will happen to good people, and justice will be served to the rest. And together with Moshiach, we will create "*Our* Perfect Life...."

Now go and play.[12]

---

12. Shmuel Pollen, "Why Does G-d Allow Suffering?" Chabad.org, https://www.chabad.org/library/article_cdo/aid/3114201/jewish/Why-Does-G-d-Allow-Suffering.htm. Used by permission of Chabad.org.

1 *My Early Life*

Edmonton

> I was a very popular girl, and had many friends.

I was born in 1952, in Edmonton, Alberta, Canada. My father, Sam Belzberg, *z"l*, was a man of his word, running his business – banking, real estate, and investments – with honesty and integrity. He traveled a lot, and when he was home, he tended to run the family like his business.

My mother, Frances, was a soft and beautiful woman. In her generation, if a woman worked outside the home, it was widely considered an embarrassment to her husband. So, she did some modeling and acting for no pay.

I am the oldest of four children. My brother Marc and sisters Wendy and Lisa are two, five, and eight years younger than me, respectively.

I can't remember much about my formative years. Either they were so bad that I don't want to remember, or – more likely – so good that they became a delightful blur and there is nothing that stands out or troubles me.

My first clear memories are from Talmud Torah School, which I attended from the first through the sixth grade. The teachers I remember include Mrs. Ely and Mrs. Lorand for English, and Mrs. Gershon and Mr. and Mrs. Levine for Hebrew. Throughout grade school, I passed English and Hebrew with honors.

I was a very popular girl and had many friends. Like so many normal children all over the world, my friends and I used to hang out during the week and have sleepovers on weekends and holidays. It was absolutely freezing in the winters – a lot of snow and a high wind chill factor. At the first snowfall, we would put the virgin snow in a bowl and pour maple syrup over it. It was like a modern-day snow cone, but without the preservatives. I did this till I got sick to my stomach. That was the end of that.

I was also very popular with the boys – maybe because during recess I used to do somersaults and twirls on the monkey bars? In the sixth grade, I had my first boyfriend, Barry Goldberg. We were together for quite a long time, but after his father died, I had no idea what to say to him. At that young age, I simply could find no way to relate to him anymore, so our special friendship petered out.

In the sixth grade, I remember my math teacher, Mrs. Walker, a stout, matronly woman who wore old-fashioned dresses and thick black oxford shoes. She had thin red hair with bald spots and a bulbous red nose streaked with purple veins. She gave me my first U (unsatisfactory) grade in math. One day when I approached her desk, she had her student book open to the IQ scores, and I saw that my score was extremely low. I was too young then to understand what an IQ score was, but knowing that my score was so low left me feeling "dumb" in too many ways. It is a stigma I carry around with me to this very day.

After grade school, I attended a local public junior high school within walking distance of my home. There were only two other Jewish girls at the school who had also studied at Talmud Torah School. One of them, Jenny Zottenberg, became my best friend. We hung out together constantly. Our school would send us home for lunch, and every day we would go to Jenny's house because it was closer to the school than mine. We would make "eggy deals" (eggs with everything under the sun in them) and eat celery and Cheez Whiz. Then, after spending nearly every day together, we would talk on the telephone after school from our homes. On the weekends, we would alternate sleeping at each other's houses.

Soon after starting public school, I had a new boyfriend, Roy Cotton. While construction work was being done in our house, Roy and I would sneak into the basement and hang out, getting away from everything and everyone for a while, and innocently "chill" together, as we used to say then.

At that time, the "in" thing among my friends was to hang out at the community center on the weekends and get drunk. My father wanted me to have nothing to do with this. He told me, "I don't want you to get drunk outside. Bring a few friends over, and I'll serve you drinks in the house." So I brought Jenny and another girl home, and my father served us vodka and orange juice, and rum and Coke. I became nauseated and vomited all over the house. I remember saying the lewdest, crudest things, and to this day, I have no idea where they came from. Suffice it to say, I was not proud of myself. From that day onward, however, I have remained unable to drink anything at all – no hard liquor and not even wine for Kiddush (the blessing over wine to sanctify the Sabbath meals).

My wise father had taught me a life lesson, although I still had many more to learn.

School days continued, and because I thought I was stupid, I barely got through. I was even caught cheating several times.

In high school, Jenny and I continued to be "besties" even though she was in the vocational training program and I was in the regular academic program. We still slept over at each other's houses every weekend and were constantly on the phone with each other when we were not in the same room.

We even sewed identical dresses for ourselves with the help of Jenny's mother. In fact, Mrs. Zottenberg ended up sewing my clothes for me, because I found sewing rather a challenge. Jenny and I would arrange to wear our matching outfits the next day at school.

Vancouver

I was dragged kicking and screaming onto the airplane.

When I turned sixteen, at the end of tenth grade, my father decided he would have better business opportunities in Vancouver, British Columbia. I, of course, had a very, very best friend and a boyfriend, neither of whom I wanted to leave. I was dragged kicking and screaming onto the airplane.

We rented a house in Vancouver while renting out our house in Edmonton, so we could easily return if my father's expectations for improving his business didn't work out. To my chagrin, it turned out to be a very profitable move. We stayed in Vancouver, joining the local Conservative synagogue.

I had been busy and popular in Edmonton, but when we first got to Vancouver, I would just sit in my room, lock my door, and cry my eyes out over my fate. However, once I met people through the synagogue and started eleventh grade at Eric Hamber School, a local public high school, I found new friends. Janice Frome was assigned to show me around the school and introduce me to everybody. After school on the first day, she took me to a park behind the school building, where nearly everyone I had met was hanging out, smoking cigarettes and marijuana. I did smell something strange, but being very innocent, I had no clue what it was. At first, having no idea about what was going on, I felt very frightened; but I soon learned that I could just hang out there without having to participate.

Janice and I soon became inseparable, and we started going out with two boys who were also friends.

Fortunately, by the end of eleventh grade, I was happily and totally assimilated into the school and into Vancouver life in general. Edmonton became a thing of my past, although I kept in touch with Jenny Zottenberg.

In the twelfth grade, I went to a concert at a different local high school, where I noticed a guy named Robert Mickelson. A friend of mine introduced us, and it was love at first sight. We immediately started dating, and thus began a wonderful, meaningful two-year relationship.

A Jewish man named Jack Diamond owned a local race track and used to hire teenagers for the summer months. To make some money of my own, I began working there as a cashier. I felt very sad to see so many very poor people spending their last dollars betting on a horse that usually lost, knowing that their money could have been put to much better use. Eventually, this became too much for me, and I left.

Anorexia Nervosa

| I did not realize what a dangerous condition this was.

Around this time, I suddenly changed my eating habits, eating only one big meal a day. One day I would consume a large bowl of fruit and yogurt; the next, I ate only a large bowl of vegetables and yogurt. Long before it was more widely recognized, I was developing the condition known as anorexia nervosa. I got down to eighty pounds and looked like a Holocaust victim. To my eyes, however, I still looked fat. I felt very light and airy. I did not realize what a dangerous condition this was.

My mother made an appointment for me at Scripps Clinic in La Jolla, California, to see a specialist in eating disorders. While we were in the waiting room, a young man started aggressively peppering me with questions: "Why do you look so emaciated?"; "Don't you ever eat anything?"; "Why don't you take care of yourself?" Thankfully the doctor removed us from this very uncomfortable situation, but the young man hit a nerve. I looked at myself more closely and started wondering, *What exactly is going on with me?*

The doctor recorded my medical history, and then we had a long chat. At the end he threatened me: "Either you shape up and start eating, or I will keep you in the hospital for six months to a year for treatment, because this could be fatal at the rate you are going." Being the warrior that I am, I said I would go home and eat. And this is indeed what I did. I slowly started eating again and nursed myself up to a healthier weight.

To this day, I believe I still carry around an anorexic mentality. Often, when I look at myself in the mirror, I see fat, even though in my head, I know I am not. The exact cause of anorexia nervosa is unknown, but it probably results from a combination of biological, psychological, and environmental factors. On the biological level, there may be genetic changes that make some people more vulnerable to developing the condition, although this is not yet clear. Some people may have a genetic tendency toward perfectionism, sensitivity, and perseverance, all traits associated with anorexia. On the psychological level, some specific character traits may also contribute to this. Young women may have obsessive-compulsive personality tendencies that make it easier for them to stick to strict diets and forgo food despite being hungry. They may have an extreme drive for perfection, which causes them to think they are never thin enough. They may have high levels of anxiety and engage in restrictive eating to reduce it.

And, of course, the environment has an impact on anorexia. Modern Western culture emphasizes thinness. Success and worthiness are often equated with being thin. Peer pressure may help fuel the desire to be thin, particularly among young girls, who are more likely to suffer from anorexia, although others can also be affected. I never did figure out in which category I fit.

2 *Young Adulthood*

The Flower Child Years

> I saw people who were living valueless, purposeless lives with nothing to look forward to other than another day of drug and sex orgies and loud rock music.

After completing high school, I enrolled in the University of British Columbia and drove back and forth from home to my studies every day in my orange stick-shift Toyota. The university had open courses, but I had no plan or focus. So I took a course called Arts 1 and basically petered away my time, taking any course that appealed to me.

The summer after that first year of "study," my high school sweetheart Robert wanted to travel with me; but I had found a new love that he couldn't relate to at all: yoga. I excelled at it and went to daily classes. Soon I had a whole new set of friends to hang out with.

Although my relationship with Robert came to an end, I soon met Craig Perkins, a redhead with a very long ponytail who was enthusiastically involved with yoga and transcendental meditation. He was a kind, sweet, gentle, spiritual person; although he was not of my faith, this didn't bother me at the time, and we moved in together.

I tried the meditation too, but it did nothing for me. Still, for Craig's sake, I just continued doing it, pretending that it was working.

In the meantime, I worked as a waitress in a vegetarian restaurant, while cultivating a little plot of organic vegetables just outside the city. I also made peanut butter balls in the basement – enlisting the help of my siblings – and tried selling them at the restaurant. The business was not much of a success, as we ended up eating most of the peanut butter balls ourselves. (I must admit they were delicious.)

Like so many around me, I was banning the bra and becoming a full-fledged flower child or hippie. While I was in the throes of my hippiedom, my mother took me to San Francisco, where it all began. I was not enthralled: I saw people who, I felt, were living valueless, purposeless lives with nothing to look forward to other than another day of drug and sex orgies and loud rock music. They took each day as it came with no goals, plans for the future, or thoughts of bringing any good into the world. It was all about "me" and how could I make myself feel good. Thinking about this woke me up: *Is this what I want my life to look like?* My conclusion was a heartfelt no.

Looking back to that time, this could have been the impetus that propelled me to start my religious lifestyle, the exact opposite of hippiedom. I remember walking into my house braless, to find my brother and a bunch of his friends in the middle of a Bible class given by Rabbi Pinchas Bak, *z"l* (the rabbi who helped my brother to become religious). My appearance had quite an effect!

One evening I went with my parents to see the musical *Fiddler on the Roof*, and the scene where one of Tevya's daughters left her family to be with her non-Jewish boyfriend had an impact on me, because there I was, living with my non-Jewish boyfriend.

My brother and two sisters had already become religious. I had taken so many journeys already, my mother suggested that I should check out my own religion, as well. I started learning with

Rabbi Hier and was soon hooked. We started learning daily along with another woman, Laura Dunner, with whom I became good friends. The distance between Craig and me grew wider and wider. At first, he followed me to synagogue on Shabbat, confiding that he might convert to Judaism; but he soon stopped pursuing me, and we broke up.

Becoming Religious

| My body and my soul glowed.

Until 1972, I was a happy, fun-loving, gregarious, outgoing flower child. This would soon change. I quickly became a full-fledged religious woman – the last one in my family. My parents never tried to follow our path and initially were angry about having to keep the house kosher – with new pots and pans, dishes, and silverware – so my siblings and I could eat there. Now I understand how threatened they must have felt. They had brought us up with good values, so why was that not enough for us? Today they are very proud of us, especially in comparison to some of their friends' children, who have overdosed on drugs, committed suicide, or done other appalling things.

Becoming a *baalat teshuvah* (a returnee to my religion), I felt ethereal, angelic, as if I were walking on clouds. My body and my soul glowed. My face shone. I found myself intoxicated with God. I walked with the Shechinah (the divine presence) at my side day and night. When I performed a mitzvah (commandment) properly, I truly felt God's love pouring down on my whole being with pride. When I did something improperly, I would feel in my heart a deep thud of fear and remorse. I was constantly striving for perfection in every aspect of religious observance. My goal was to make His will my will.

After maintaining this level of relationship with Judaism for a while, I felt that God had shown me where I was going and how high I could reach. But then I felt Him slipping away. *No, wait – please don't leave me … I'm not ready yet.* Now I felt that He was telling me that I needed to work on my own, make my own progress and carve out my own path rather than rely completely on Him to show me the way.

With this realization, I felt Him letting go of my hand, although I still felt His presence, as if He was telling me, *I'll still be by your side, and if you need My help, I will gladly help you.* I felt a little bereft and lonely, but soon realized that from now on, my Yiddishkeit (Jewishness) would be what I made of it myself. Years later, I would hear Rabbi Noach Orlowek say, "God only takes away what he gave you – what you earn yourself He doesn't take away."

As a newly religious but not very knowledgeable woman, I decided to attend Stern College (a college for religious Jewish women in New York) for a year, focusing solely on Judaic studies. I totally immersed myself in my newfound love. Everything about the experience was awesome. I had inspiring teachers who fed my thirst for knowledge. One of them, Rabbi Avi Weiss, had a very big influence on me. I would sit in the front row in his class right in front of him. To this day I can still see him in his stocking feet jumping up and down giving over his Bible class with such enthusiasm and such love penetrating to the depth of my soul. He was also the first person to call me by my Hebrew name, influencing some of my friends, who till this day still call me Rifka. Forty-seven years later, Rabbi Weiss and I are still in touch. We have a special place for each other in our hearts.

However, as the second half of this enchanted year began, my handwriting suddenly became totally illegible, for no reason that

I could ascertain. My voice inexplicably became monotonic, also apparently without reason. I started gaining weight, which at least I could attribute to my nightly raid of brownies from the vending machine. Not only was I baffled by all these changes, some of which were inexplicable, but I also became depressed.

I felt God had made me ill. If I wanted to be cynical, I could wonder whether this was my reward for becoming religious, but... I am not going to go there. I was overwhelmed by these changes, which interfered with my studies and challenged my relationship with God.

I became self-obsessed. Perhaps this was understandable under the circumstances, but it certainly was far from ideal. All I wanted once again was that visceral feeling of love from God and being in His tight, all-encompassing hug, as I first felt when my religious journey began. I ran after every mitzvah possible wholeheartedly to try to change the decree, but after a while, I came to the realization that this was not working. From then on I had to push myself extremely hard to get out of bed every morning and just keep afloat. God and His mitzvot were not on my radar at all. Anything I did religiously was just serendipitous. What I did not realize was that you can serve and come close to God in whatever situation you find yourself in; but I was not there yet.

At that time, my brother Marc was studying at Yeshiva University (a college for religious Jewish men) in New York. Soon an opportunity arose to hear him speak at a convention of the Orthodox Union in Florida about the positive effect that the organization's youth group, the National Conference of Synagogue Youth (NCSY), had had on his life. NCSY was dedicated to connecting Jewish teens with their Jewish tradition.

The trip to Florida was fateful. Not only did I enjoy the privilege of hearing Marc speak so inspiringly and enthusiastically, but I also met my future husband, Harvey Tannenbaum. He was at the convention as an officer of the Orthodox Union. Spying each other from a distance, we made our approaches and began chatting. Harvey was a very active member of NCSY, and every weekend he traveled throughout the West Coast on missions, trying to help lost youth reclaim their Jewish heritage. We discovered that we had an earlier connection, as he had shown my brother how to lay tefillin (phylacteries) when Marc had started becoming religious.

After the convention, Harvey returned to Los Angeles, and I went back to my studies in New York at Stern. The strong connection had been forged. Long before the age of computers and emails, we kept in touch through daily phone calls and snail-mailed letters. Despite the challenges the distance presented, we strengthened our deep bond.

Harvey had campaigned for Richard Nixon's reelection and was subsequently invited to his second inauguration. Harvey invited me to be his date. How exciting! He picked me up at Stern College, creating quite a commotion as all the girls came out of their dorm rooms, like a swarm of ants, to see who my new heartthrob was. We spent Shabbat in Silver Spring, Maryland, staying with two different families within walking distance of each other. Over Shabbat, we could connect on a more personal level. He was a very charming, charismatic, personable, and handsome man.

After Shabbat was out, we set out for the inaugural ball, Harvey in a rented tuxedo and me in my gown. It was a thrill just being there with a crowd of famous people (not that I had heard of any of them, having been so sheltered), all dressed to the nines and oozing in jewels. And, no, I was not at all jealous, being the simple person that I am; nonetheless, it was a little impressive to be an unworldly bystander.

Even at the ball, Harvey and I respected a proper level of modesty, and although there was mixed dancing, we remained just observers, since mixed dancing is frowned upon in Jewish religious circles. The whole experience was quite a sight to see, although, in all honesty, it could just as easily have been a sight to be missed in terms of any deeper meaning. Still, it was a very exciting evening, and on Sunday morning we each returned to our respective homes in New York and Los Angeles.

Once again we resumed our long-distance relationship until the end of my school year. At that point, I decided to go stay with my grandmother in Los Angeles for the summer. (Surprise, surprise!) I enrolled in a course in abnormal psychology at UCLA, but the true purpose of my stay in Los Angeles was to be with Harvey. He was also taking some summer-school classes, so we hung out together on campus and then spent most evenings at his house or my grandmother's, or we would go out to eat or see a movie. We were quite inseparable.

One day that summer, as I was walking out of my class, down the grassy path of the campus, my right leg began to kick my left ankle. Since this only happened occasionally, I thought that perhaps I was unconsciously adopting some of the symptoms of the cases that I was learning about in my psych class. Perhaps when the course ended, the kicking would go away. To my horror, however, the kicking started to occur with every step I took, and after the course ended, the kicking continued.

At the end of the summer, I returned to Vancouver and tried to figure out how to fill my days constructively while waiting for Harvey to propose... One night, I was in the kitchen with my mother, helping her prepare a salad. When she spoke to me, I suddenly found myself unable to answer her. My lips were frozen and would not move. When I finally managed to speak, my words came out slurred: they were unintelligible. My whole family thought it was a joke and started imitating and making fun of me. This continued and became more intense until they realized I was not joking. My father, who did not take failure very well, as he never failed, found it particularly disturbing not to be able to understand his own daughter. Ultimately, he became very frustrated and, because of his distress, lost all patience with me. My mother, on the other hand, listened and listened till she understood what I said. I guess this is a mother's job.

Now unable to speak, with my feet still kicking, I realized it was time to see my physician. He had no idea what was wrong with me, so he sent me to several neurologists for a slew of tests. The results all came back indicating that my health was normal. My physician reiterated that I was in perfectly good health. Nobody could identify the cause of my problems, so they attributed it to conversion hysteria – today this is called conversion disorder – connecting my symptoms with my newfound interest in religion and my strong reactions to the suffering of the Jewish people throughout history.

My doctors referred me to a psychiatrist. Twice a week, over the course of about a month, I sat in his office, where he would converse with me, trying to figure out the root of the problem. I simply bawled my eyes out. I could not understand why I was there. To me, it seemed perfectly obvious that the problem causing my suffering was physical and not psychological. I was totally sane.

In the end, I simply stopped going to the therapist, convinced that it was a complete waste of time, and that I was no closer to discovering the root of the two debilitating problems plaguing me every second of the day. Back in Los Angeles, Harvey kept up with what was happening, but did not know how to help me. He trusted that I knew what was right for me and supported my decision to stop going to therapy.

My Hand in Marriage

> We were convinced that changing
> my life would change my luck.

While anxiously awaiting Harvey's proposal, I took a typing course. My typewriter became my voice, as I could now express myself through writing. It became an important component in my life.

Finally, Harvey asked my father for my hand in marriage. My father interrogated him, making sure he understood what he was taking on, since I was ill. Harvey was sure. My problem had been diagnosed as hysteria, so we were convinced that changing my life would change my luck. We believed that starting a new life together and moving to a new city would surely cure my "hysteria" and help me snap out of it. We were in for a surprise.

We married on June 18, 1974, the first Orthodox Jewish wedding to be held at the Hyatt Regency in Vancouver. The next day, we flew to Los Angeles for the *sheva berachot* (a week of meals and blessings according to traditional Jewish custom). Was our plane's engine trouble a good omen or a bad omen? I was uncertain.

The afternoon before the first of the blessings, I bought a very ugly light blue turban – matching my dress for the occasion – to cover my hair in accordance with strict Jewish laws of modesty pertaining to married women. Covering my head was entirely new to me, and I felt very proud to take on this special mitzvah. A woman's hair is her "crowning glory," so it felt right to save this just for my husband. Today, I have progressed from that first ugly turban to fancy, colorful hats and scarves tied in unusual ways.

In Los Angeles, we soon moved into our first rented apartment. My mother helped; well, she decorated it for us. I did not care, because soon after the *sheva berachot*, I was preoccupied with physical problems and feeling miserable. Day in and day out, I would sit in a corner with my back against the wall, wearing my husband's UCLA shorts, pinned at the sides because they were too big for me, and his large white undershirt – backwards, because it was too low in the front. Occasionally, I would muster up some energy to try to clean something – a dish or a part of the floor. Then I would return to my little corner and brood.

3 *The Epitome of Health*

Misdiagnosis and Diagnosis

> *There seemed to be a dissonance here.*

Basically, I was nonfunctional. I felt as if a hose in my gut was siphoning off every bit of strength I had, which wasn't much. It tore Harvey apart to see me like this, but he continued to feel totally helpless and was unable to help me. We spent our "honeymoon" at the Scripps Clinic, still searching for answers, being told the exact same thing: all the test results were normal, and all I had was hysteria.

Torah Judaism is a religion. It is truth. It is about having a personal one-on-one deep, spiritual soul relationship with God. It is about refining one's character, living a morally upstanding life, and committing acts of kindness. Yet ostensibly, observing it was causing me to be hysterical to the point of completely disability. There seemed to be a dissonance here. To my mind, this religion has so many laudable qualities that just did not fit the diagnosis of hysteria. Nonetheless, everyone was against me: the doctors were so arrogant that they were unable to admit their utter inability to identify my condition. They therefore felt a need to blame it on something, anything…so hysteria it was.

Here was my thought process: If it truly was hysteria, then

there must have been something in my previous environment that disagreed with me. So moving to a new city, away from my family, making a bunch of new friends, would put an end to the hysteria. The doctors suggested that I participate in an adult development group at UCLA for people with psychiatric problems. So we returned to Los Angeles, where I was to start my life as a married woman, going to a crazy house every day.

There I met my psychiatrist, Dr. Walter Kaye. I was reticent about the whole situation and felt I would not fit into the group with all their serious psychological issues. I could neither walk nor talk: What was so hard to understand? This was not in my mind. In fact, my mantra was "This is not in my mind," because the whole world was telling me that it was.

Dr. Markham, an acquaintance of Dr. Kaye's and connected to UCLA, started discussing my bizarre case. He suggested that I go into the hospital for some more testing. So, there I was again, going through the whole gamut of neurological tests available at that time, only to be told once again that I was the epitome of health, who just so happened to be unable to walk or talk.

Dr. Markham had left me in the hands of interns and disappeared. I was upset with him for decades. In 2013, just when I had worked up the courage to tell him how disappointed I was, he died.

Back to square one. I left the group and continued my quest to find an answer. I found another neurologist, Dr. Andrea Nash, who examined me. After more tests, one finally came back positive for Wilson's disease, which involves a copper ring around the eye. While I was sitting in Dr. Nash's office reviewing the diagnosis, the lab called and told her that they had given her the wrong results. She told me that she was convinced that I had a physical illness – although she could not identify it – and referred me to her superior, Dr. John Menkes (who has since died as well).

I tried to make an appointment, but Dr. Menkes was booked up for months, with his only opening on Saturday – the Jewish

Shabbat (Sabbath), when religious Jews may not travel or do any creative work. I consulted with my rabbi, and he said that I could walk there. It took two miles and two hours of my feet kicking each other down the street to reach his office. After examining me, Dr. Menkes diagnosed me with a rare neurological condition called dystonia musculorum deformans.

Finally, it was confirmed: I was *not* crazy, and it was not hysteria. I truly was ill. My initial indescribable elation at finally finding a medical reason for my condition was shattered when the doctor proceeded to tell me how rare it is, that there is no known cause, and, thus, no known treatment or cure.

Poor Harvey! All his hopes, dreams, and visions, all his goals and fantasies for a new marriage and a new life were obliterated instantly with the word *dystonia*. He was totally shattered, and so was I. On the one hand, it was a huge relief that I was not suffering from hysteria; on the other hand, it was devastating to know that we would have to deal with a chronic, incurable illness…possibly, for the rest of our lives.

In the dark, abstruse world of dystonia, "treatment" is a euphemism for experimentation. I became a guinea pig and was given a wide range of medications to try to alleviate my symptoms. Not one helped; in fact, most of them caused debilitating side effects that were usually much worse than any possible benefits – which, in my case, numbered zero. Starting a medication, waiting for it to reach the optimal dosage level at which the desired effects should be felt, only to find out that they did not happen. And so, on to the next, and the next after that… Many times, unable to endure the horrible side effects, I was forced to meet Dr. Menkes in the emergency room at the local hospital. This process taught me the gift of patience. I can think of numerous more positive ways to learn this.

One drug that was prescribed, 5-HTP, was not FDA approved, and I received it in powder form. I had to spend two hours every day filling up seventy gel capsules. I began to experience excruciating pain in my body and was admitted to the hospital under the care of Dr. Sue, my general physician at that time. I had had the foresight to bring with me all the medications that I was taking. When the pain failed to subside, the doctors discovered that the 5-HTP was tainted. We eventually sued the company that had manufactured it, and after a few years, we received some monetary compensation.

The pain did not ease until the doctor prescribed prednisone. It was simply remarkable, imbuing me with so much unlimited energy that I was unable to sleep and stayed up all night painting velvet pictures that came in a kit. Once a week, I would see a psychiatrist, Dr. Barnett Malin. He could not cure me, but every time I arrived at his office, I felt that I was entering a safe, nonjudgmental haven, where there was a receptive ear. There I felt that I could cry, vent, rage at my illness and the unfairness of it all, and discuss my frustrations concerning my unfulfilled goals, wishes, and dreams.

The Dystonia Medical Research Foundation

> How horrifying it must be to see one's child suffering right before one's very eyes, with no solution at hand.

When we finally received my diagnosis, my father was at his wits' end as to how to help me. How horrifying it must be to see one's child suffering right before one's very eyes, with no solution at hand. Unfortunately, money cannot buy health, but it can be used to do other things. After finally learning the name of my rare ailment, discovering that it had neither a known cause nor a known treatment, my father spoke to my doctor about starting the Dystonia Medical Research Foundation to fund serious studies on the disease. My parents set up two committees: one for scientific research, and the other – the volunteer board – for raising funds.

The scientific board first met in September 1975. The eight doctors involved began a lively discussion about how best to go about researching this mysterious disease.

My father also took Dr. Menkes to Washington, DC, to confer with the National Institutes of Health, in hopes of partnering with the government researchers in some way. At that time, they told us that they only knew of approximately three cases of dystonia in North America, and it was not worth their while to become involved. Undeterred, my father thanked them and went his merry way to do it alone. At a subsequent scientific board meeting, which my parents attended, one doctor thought he might be on to something, but would not share it until after he had published it. Dad told the doctor that he had to realize that this board was put together precisely for identifying the disease, finding a treatment, and – eventually – a cure. This meant that everyone was supposed to be sharing information and ideas. Perhaps, my father suggested, this voluntary board was not for him? The doctor was asked to leave.

Since my parents were personally funding the board, they sat in on all the grant reviews. We did not realize that we were setting a precedent of nonprofessionals sitting with professionals; in fact, this is unique to the Dystonia Foundation, and my parents continued this practice.

In the beginning, Dr. Menkes in Los Angeles and his assistant, Nancy Harris, acted as the central office before the foundation became accredited. Eventually, we decided to add an official executive director in Vancouver, who worked out of my father's office. Lois Raphael took up this post and drew up pamphlets about dystonia in both French and English, for circulation to doctors' offices throughout Canada. We hoped to alert doctors to the symptoms, thereby possibly saving people from going through the trauma that I had experienced.

Through the efforts of both the Los Angeles and Canadian offices, and as more doctors became aware of dystonia in its myriad forms, both the scientific board and the volunteer board grew. Through the volunteer board, we were able to raise funds for research.

It became clear after some ten years of building the foundation that we needed one central head office with an executive director who had a history of working with other medical foundations and knowledge about fundraising. We eventually opened this office in Chicago in June 2002 with professional staff. Janet Hieshetter was at the helm.

The foundation has now been in existence for over forty years. When its work began, there were only three known dystonia patients in North America. Under the guidance of the executive office, it has since identified 300,000 sufferers. Ironically, the foundation has helped many people, but not the one for whom it was created – me: the form of dystonia that I have does not fit into any of the recognized categories. As a result, after forty-five years, I still have no precise diagnosis. I used to joke with my father that he would have to start a new foundation once I get my primary diagnosis. I am confident that one day, hopefully soon, I will be helped by medical advancements, or the Messiah will come first.

4 Building Our Family

Life in Los Angeles

> We assumed that Harvey would just get back together with his regular group of friends, and that I would become involved with their wives.

When we had first arrived in Los Angeles, we assumed that Harvey would just get back together with his regular group of friends, and that I would become involved with their wives. This was not to be. We were pariahs. No one could understand how such a handsome, popular, sought-after young man could have married a woman who was so ill she was unable to communicate verbally or move around. No one knew how to relate to me.

Harvey was totally devastated by the situation. He was angry at God, Who made me ill. We were both suffering and grieving the idyllic honeymoon period we had expected this first year of marriage to be.

After months of inaction and misery, I was fed up and determined to do something productive. I enrolled at UCLA to study for a bachelor's degree in psychology. Among the many courses I took was a statistics class in which I had to work with white rats. I was petrified of them at first, but after a while, they became my friends, and I named them Sarah and Leah. In the past I had always had an affinity for animals, and Sarah and Leah helped return it to me. I think I connected with them – and all animals in general – because one does not need to talk to them. All one must do is play with them and caress them – just give them unconditional love. At the end of the course, I even took Sarah and Leah home.

Another favorite course of mine was a behavioral modification lab taught by the late Dr. Ivar Lovaas, who discovered the use of behavior modification techniques with autistic children. I worked with a pair of autistic twins who happened to share my birthday. My cousin David Cooper built a wooden toy house to help me with my work, and the twins and I played with it, using miniature people, beds, house and kitchen supplies, and the like.

I found that I liked working with special needs children. It seemed to me that children under the age of five had no trouble understanding me. I thought that the reason for this might be that they do not yet have an established language pattern.

After earning my bachelor's degree in psychology, I worked at a clinic, treating another autistic child. Thinking that working with special needs children was my calling, I enrolled at Pacific Oaks College in Pasadena to obtain certification to teach special education. I would drive an hour in each direction every day for my studies. When I had already completed 88 percent of the course work, I learned that one of the requirements for receiving this degree was teaching in a regular classroom. With my speech problem, there was no way I could teach a classroom of twenty or so rowdy students. Not one to be deterred from achieving my goal, I petitioned the college to exempt me from this requirement, given my special circumstances; they denied my request. In the end, I wrote a thesis on dystonia and received a master's degree in human development (whatever that is). I later realized that I had not learned any real teaching skills, and most probably I would not have known what to do had I been placed in a classroom. In the end, I realized that what had happened was for the good.

Still searching for something to do, I thought that my love of clothes and my knack for putting them together in very interesting ways could provide me with some direction: perhaps I could design windows for clothing stores. I applied to fashion design school, although I had neither a talent for drawing nor any desire to design clothes. At the end of my first year, the people in charge of the program told me that because of my physical condition, designing windows would not be safe for me, because the work involved climbing ladders, moving mannequins, and other such activities.

Once again, unwilling to be thwarted, I petitioned the administration for an exemption, and once again my petition was rejected. Trying very hard not to feel frustrated, I had to say to myself over and over that these setbacks were from God, these places were simply not right for me, and that I just needed to keep searching for the right fit.

Going through piles of catalogues for study and courses, I came across a jewelry-making course that looked interesting. I decided to give it a try. Mind you, I did not have a creative bone in my body... or so I thought. I fell in love both with the entire process of jewelry making and with the results.

The teacher of the class told us to go to Winagura, a local whole-sale bead store, to purchase some supplies. Not knowing that at a wholesale bead store, you buy the beads and then leave, I sat down at a table in the store and began making necklaces with the beads I had chosen. I continued doing this for the next two years. I was lucky that Marion and Murray Winagura, the proprietors of the store, were quite fond of me, so it was fine with them that I had set up a workshop there. As I wandered about, I would observe everything around me and imagine ways in which to transform designs that I liked into necklaces by placing beads on a wire. I amassed a vast collection of unique necklaces but, having only one neck, I thought I should try to sell some.

Well, that did not happen. It was not easy to find a market of very gutsy people willing to wear one of my pieces. Stores would not take them because I did not take orders for repeated designs: everything I made was one of a kind. Deciding that I would be my own walking advertisement, I kept changing necklaces a few times a day and walking around with them. And sure enough, on a few occasions women bought necklaces off my neck. Around September 1981, I was substituting for aides for special needs classes in the Los Angeles school district. This involved getting a call at 6 a.m. from someone who would tell me which school to go to. It did not make for an easy life. I was sick of therapy and of trying medications that did not work. My soul was crying out for something, but I did not know what.

Until October 12, 1985. It was Shabbat Bereishit, when the reading of Genesis (the first of the five books of the Bible) begins in synagogue. We walked to synagogue, taking our usual "scenic" route down all the alleys and lanes overflowing with garbage cans, where nary a soul would tread, and where I therefore could not be seen.

Reading about Eve, the mother of all human life, I realized that a major part of a woman's role in the Jewish religion is having children, to perpetuate the Jewish people, to teach them the proper direction in life, and to raise them to be loyal servants of God. I experienced an epiphany that I did not want to miss out on this holy privilege.

My doctors told me that my condition was genetic and that there was a 50 percent chance of having a child with dystonia. They advised me very strongly against having children: I could barely take care of myself, so how would I be able to take care of a sick child? With fear and trepidation, and the doctors' words ringing in my ears on the one hand, and on my other, stronger hand – confident in my

faith that God knows what is best for me and that He would give
me what I needed and what I could handle – I made up my mind to
pursue my quest to become a mother. I decided that, after thirteen
years of trying different useless medications to try to heal my illness,
Harvey and I should discuss the pros and cons. As we both wanted
a child, we decided that I would stop taking my medicines and take
a leap of faith. I became pregnant immediately. I stopped subbing
in the school district because I did not want my fetus to be exposed
to such a depressing scene, even indirectly.

The pregnancy was not easy for me. It was difficult to carry forty
pounds of extra weight. Strangely, however, it became physically
easier for me to speak: my lips seemed to be looser, although my
voice still sounded the same – unintelligible.

I was under the care of excellent doctors and had regular monthly
checkups. When I went to my doctor's office at Cedar Sinai Hospital
for the seventh monthly checkup, he told me that I must remain
there in a hospital bed with a monitor attached to my abdomen,
because the fetus was in constant distress. I was shocked and asked
why I could not just confine myself to bed rest in my own home.
One of the doctors on the team knew me very well and understood
that if I went home, I would not be able to sit still for one minute.

So there I was, stuck in the hospital for two months. At least I had
numerous visitors. Once, a friend even took me on an outing in a
wheelchair: we went into the gift shop, where there was a full-length
mirror. This was the first time I had seen my body in a month.

I remember that, as a teenager, I used to think that pregnant
women were so fat and ugly that they should be confined some-
where out of sight until they gave birth. Now, however, I was awed
by the changes in my belly; how big and round and beautiful it
looked. It made me wonder why there are no mirrors in hospitals.
Perhaps it is because ill people do not want to see the alterations
in themselves, going from once-robust individuals to a new, frail,
frightening state.

At that point, only my doctor knew the sex of the child. Harvey and I did not want to know in advance. I was due around Passover, so if it was a boy, my family from out of town would have to scramble for accommodations in order to be at the circumcision ceremony and for Passover. My father tried to cajole the doctor into telling him the gender of the fetus so that he could make plans, but my doctor maintained strict confidentiality.

Orit's Birth

| She was our light.

It was Shabbat Hagadol, the Sabbath before Passover. The monitor showed that my baby was in fetal distress, so they wheeled me to the gynecology ward. The doctor came running into my room, put an oxygen mask on me, and broke my waters, and then gave me oxytocin to try to induce labor. A lovely nurse who lived in my mother-in-law's building stayed with me until I went down to the operating room. My husband was also with me.

The oxytocin was not working, and the baby was increasingly suffering from distress, so they rushed me down to the operating room for an emergency cesarean section. I was given a local anesthetic, and a mirror was placed in a position where I could watch the operation. Not a pretty sight, but a beautiful outcome: a beautiful baby girl with ten fingers and ten toes, and all the rest of the necessary accoutrements.

She was born that Shabbat, weighing in at 6 lb., 13 oz. (corresponding to the 613 commandments in the Torah). We named her Orit Channah. Orit (*light* in Hebrew) because she was our light, and Channah after my father-in-law's sister.

I stayed in the hospital for a week because I had an infection.

We had a woozy, brief Seder in my room, just Harvey, Orit, and me. When the time finally came to return home and settle in with our new baby, I needed full-time help. Harvey had been interviewing women sent by an agency. Eventually, he found someone he thought would be suitable. I was in bed nursing when he walked in with a stocky, middle-aged woman named Zoila. She was from El Salvador, and I liked her immediately.

We hired Zoila to take charge of the house – all the standard chores of cooking, cleaning, laundry, and so on, in which I had no interest at all. My job was to look after my baby…or so I thought.

Every time I picked Orit up to hold her, she would scream. Granted, I wasn't the gentlest picker-upper, given my disability, but I was thrown by her screaming. And each time she screamed, it was Zoila to the rescue – constantly. It got to the point where Orit only wanted Zoila and would not let me near her. Zoila had to put her down for a nap, read her a book, feed her, play with her, take her for a walk, give her a bath, and put her to bed.

With no malice on Zoila's part, she slowly wormed her way into my baby's heart, until there was no longer anyone else in Orit's world but Zoila – and perhaps Harvey, a little. Harvey did not see the problem till Orit wanted nothing to do with him either. The woman I had welcomed into my house to run it literally – if unintentionally – stole my baby away from me spiritually, emotionally, mentally, and physically, all within the confines of my own home and before my very eyes.

I was not going to take this lying down, so I brought in a procession of child therapists to observe the interactions among Orit, Zoila, and me. Not one of them could provide an explanation, but they did suggest that I should stay with Zoila while she did everything, so that at least I would be present.

My only advantage over Zoila was that I was nursing Orit. I became depressed and thought that I needed to start taking medication again. I have no idea where that came from, because no medication had ever helped me; nonetheless, once again I started trying different medicines...which prevented me from nursing. Gone was my last vestige of connection to Orit. I was very jealous of Zoila and hated the sight of her, but I still needed her.

Not satisfied with the child development specialists' suggestions, I decided to consult with a specialist in the field of mother-child interactions. This entailed a two-hour drive, and, not knowing the highway system, I got totally lost. When I finally arrived, only fifteen minutes of my appointment were left. As Orit screamed the whole time, we had no chance even to talk. At least the therapist witnessed part of what I was going through.

In the end, I stopped consulting with all the different therapists, because they were no help at all. They all concluded that Orit sensed I was different and that because this disturbed her, she just wanted to be with someone who was "normal" (whatever that is).

When I first developed dystonia symptoms, I was constantly thinking, *When will this go away so I can get back to normal?* Eventually I realized that when you are faced with a test, that difficult way of living every day *is* normal.

Fortunately, our baby flourished and reached all the expected milestones at the appropriate times. When the time arrived for her to start kindergarten, she attended Hillel Hebrew Academy, where she liked her teacher and had many friends. To my dismay, however, she was embarrassed to bring her friends home, because her mother had some issues. To remedy this situation, I decided to hold dance and art classes at my house. I hired teachers and all Orit's friends' mothers brought their children over to participate. My plan was a success.

We also threw lavish American-style birthday parties for her and her friends (as was the trend in those days). I remember one in particular: We hired a man to bring horses and a whole menagerie of different animals to our house. Orit dressed up as a cowgirl, and everyone took turns riding up and down the block on the ponies. What a sight that was for all the neighbors.

After Orit finished kindergarten, it was clear to me that Zoila had to go. Both she and Orit were very sad, and Orit's unrelenting tears only stopped after many hours. Then she really started to give me trouble: she began kicking me, pulling my hair, picking at my skin, and more; so off we went to yet another child specialist at UCLA, Dr. Kula. It was a fifteen-minute drive, and Orit cried every time we went there. She complained that the drive was too long, and that she got carsick. Harvey would have to pick her up, kicking and screaming, and put her in the car.

These visits were not very helpful either. No one could get to the root of the problem that she had with me. In hindsight, I think she just wanted a regular, ordinary mom like all her friends had. This was emotionally devastating for me. To have waited thirteen years to have a child and then be rejected by her was totally distressing. However, after seeing the respect with which my friends and neighbors in the community treated me, she finally realized that there was something special about her mother. We were able to build a relationship from this.

In 1990, I began experiencing severe neck pain. A neck doctor gave me cortisone shots and medicine against the pain, but this was only a temporary and unsatisfactory Band-Aid. After obtaining a second opinion, it was decided that I needed disc surgery. Dr. Duncan McBride performed the procedure at the UCLA Medical Center in September 1990. The scalpel penetrated my neck, and I now bear a little scar there to show for it. Thankfully, the surgery was successful and gave me relief.

In August 1993, I went to Israel for my nephew's bar mitzvah. I had a feeling that I was pregnant, and a blood test confirmed it. When I experienced a little spotting, I was checked into Hadassah Hospital on Mount Scopus Hospital overnight. The hospital stay was a little traumatic because there was a large lizard crawling on the floor and up my bedpost... In the morning, I was fine and was discharged from the hospital. Back home after the celebration, when I went in for my eleventh-week checkup, the doctor did an ultrasound but could not hear any heartbeat. The doctor left the room – I assume to compose himself – before walking back in and pronouncing my baby dead. I had a D&C (dilation and curettage) procedure the next day.

Such an experience can be simultaneously devastating and a blessing. Devastating because a life that had been inside of me had died, although it was too early for me to have felt real movement. I was more devastated for Orit's sake, because it was the loss of her sibling: Who knew whether there would be another chance? Nonetheless it was also a blessing, because a miscarriage meant that the child probably was not healthy. I know that I could not have handled taking care of an ill child, and could not have borne my baby's suffering.

During all those years in Los Angeles, one of my favorite activities was working as a *balanit*, a woman who helps other women prepare for and immerse in the mikveh, the Jewish ritual bath. I would work every other Friday night, alternating with another woman because the two of us lived closest to the mikveh. I couldn't work there during the week because I wouldn't have been able to call the rabbi if a question should arise (on Friday night, Shabbat, use of the phone is not permitted, so I was spared this task). My disability limits what I can do to serve the community, but I realized that this would be a viable way to contribute. In this way I was able to help women become ready to reunite intimately with their husbands. All sorts of interesting women visited the mikveh. Some were not Orthodox and didn't know all the laws, but continued using the mikveh because it was part of their tradition.

Before entering a mikveh, a woman should be completely clean, with short fingernails and no nail polish or makeup. One Friday night a woman drove up in her car (the driving already being a violation of Sabbath laws), beautifully coiffed, all decked out with nail polish and makeup. I was totally aghast and did not know what to do. I quickly got on my Shabbat-adapted scooter and drove to the nearest rabbi, to ask him for advice. An entire comedy of errors ensued as I struggled to make myself understood; the bottom line was that he said I needed to find a non-Jewish woman to draw a bath, remove her makeup and nail polish, and cut her nails. (As a Jew, I was forbidden to do these things, because it was already Shabbat.)

Where was I going to find such a person? Fortunately, there was a non-kosher seafood restaurant next to the mikveh. I walked in and spotted a waitress. Through another comedy of errors I beckoned her to the mikveh and gestured what I needed her to do. I can only imagine what she thought – *these crazy Orthodox Jews* – but she did it willingly and graciously. It was a night I will never forget: the desire of the secular woman to be immersed, the support of total strangers, and my ability to assist a woman despite my physical challenges. Maybe because of my physical challenges I was particularly eager to help. I know what it means to be a burden, and what it means to have to get people to go out of their way to help. Furthermore, I know how important it can be to a woman to be immersed in the mikveh, whatever the circumstances.

My disabilities taught me to persevere in my attempt to help people. I am very proud to have been one of the many *balaniyot* who simply want to help others perform a mitzvah.

Since our marriage, my husband worked on several projects to try to make a living. At one point, he and a partner would bring Israeli singers to Los Angeles to perform in concerts. Although he went to law school, he did not pass the bar exam. He tried his hand at hotel and property management, and eventually opened four kosher restaurants, one with Mexican cuisine, one a deli, and two pizzerias.

He was one of the pioneers of good kosher food, and his restaurants were very successful; but in the end, his success was also his undoing. He decided to open two more restaurants in a different area of Los Angeles and took on a partner to do so. Unhappily, this person's dishonesty undermined all of my husband's work, and Harvey was forced to declare bankruptcy.

What seemed like a setback at first became a great opportunity for us, because it made us realize that we could now move to Israel. (Remember that adage we had invoked years earlier when we first got married: change your place, change your luck?) Harvey's sister and my brother were already there, so we would not be alone: having family members already living in Israel helps make the transition much easier. We were able to use the money we had received from our court case to help us make the move.

We packed up our large house and, with one daughter in tow, boarded a plane on June 18, 1994, the day after O. J. Simpson's notorious car chase, when he was accused of killing his ex-wife. What an auspicious departure!

Looking back on twenty-five years of life in Los Angeles, I can identify certain major landmarks:

1. My unexplained illness becoming more pronounced
2. Receiving the devastating diagnosis of dystonia
3. Giving birth to Orit and trying to win her heart – which consumed my life
4. Receiving my bachelor's degree in psychology
5. Receiving my master's degree in human development
6. Finding my passion – jewelry making
7. Working as a *balanit* in the mikveh
8. Chilling with my friends who had the patience to overlook my illness and get to my very essence

For me, "chilling" connotes a very relaxed environment with friends bantering back and forth, but chilling with my friends was very intense. It took very deep concentration to try to read my lips and decipher what I was trying to say. It might have been difficult, but these were my true friends, and they remain so to this day.

The Move to Israel

> As soon as we landed, I felt a
> peace and contentment that I had
> finally arrived in the place where
> all Jews should be.

Our flight to Israel was long but exciting, as we were filled with anticipation of starting a new life in our homeland. As soon as we landed, I felt a peace and contentment that I had finally arrived in the place where all Jews should be, the Land of Israel.

My brother and some of his friends met us at the airport. We rented an apartment in Jerusalem's Katamon neighborhood, near my brother and the Horev School, where we wanted Orit to study. We had heard that they had a very good counselor there, Mrs. Rachel Namburg, who helps new immigrants adjust to school and a new language. Having not seen our apartment before, we received quite a shock when we got there and found that it was a little hole in the wall compared to our house in Los Angeles. I helped myself adjust by telling myself that we were giving up our materialistic desires for a more spiritual life in the Holy Land. I was busy getting Orit adjusted and getting to know where the amenities were. I still had to struggle with not being able to talk or walk, but at least now I was experiencing these problems in our homeland.

Eventually, the lease on our apartment ran out, and we found another one in the same area – just as small. We were busy unpacking and getting to know the area, even though it was not much different from where we had been before. There was a storage area behind the living room with a large window. Through the glass, we saw a bird sitting on its nest of eggs. When our cleaner, Tzila, saw this, she claimed that it was an omen for a new child. Little did she know, but at age forty-two, I was pregnant with my second child.

Nechama's Birth

> The fact of her birth was a comfort for me.

Since the move to Israel, I had been conferring with my former neurologists from Los Angeles, along with the new doctor I had found in Israel, Dr. Avinoam Reches. Finally, when I was forty, I heard from them that they did not believe that my illness was genetic. Nevertheless, this was a high-risk pregnancy, and I was fortunate to find a remarkable, angelic doctor, Dr. Simcha Yagel, who had been recommended by Dr. Larry Platt, my doctor in Los Angeles. As with my first pregnancy, I gained forty pounds, making it very difficult for me to move around.

I wanted to deliver this baby naturally, so on July 18, 1995, I entered the hospital. The staff attached a monitor to me, with a slow drip of Pitocin to induce labor. Suddenly, the monitors started beeping very loudly. The nurse called for the doctor, as she discerned fetal distress. Despite my hopes of delivering this baby naturally, once again I underwent an emergency cesarean section. This time, I was put under general anesthesia. Yet again, my dream of having my baby placed on my chest after birth was frustrated; but the results were wonderful, no matter how difficult the process. We named her Nechama Adeena. Nechama means *comfort* in Hebrew, and this was the perfect name for her, because the fact of her birth was a comfort for me. The name Adeena was in memory of my maternal grandmother Dena.

Orit and Harvey were thrilled by the new arrival. Finally, Orit had a sibling. She was too old to be jealous, even though the baby usurped her place. She became Nechama's "second mother," helping as much as possible given her busy schedule, and enjoying every minute of it. Harvey was thrilled because he had another daughter.

I hired a girl, Avigail Zev, to help me take care of Nechama. I tried to nurse the baby, but had little milk. I became a little depressed, but is that not normal after giving birth? I was busy taking care of both my baby and Orit, getting her to various afterschool activities. My neck was bothering me again, and I found out I needed further disc surgery. I went into surgery in a Tel Aviv hospital, expecting to feel relief from my neck pain. What I did not expect was to lose the use of my right arm. We were all a little unnerved by this eventuality, and I needed help to do various things, such as get dressed, for about six months. Because of my illness, I qualified for full-time help from a caregiver, and we received this assistance from a woman from the Philippines. Slowly but surely, with physical therapy, daily exercises, and time, I regained the use of my arm.

Simcha's Birth

| He is filled with joy.

Two years later, at the age of forty-four, I became pregnant again. I was thrilled at the news, as were Harvey and Orit. I was worried about the risk of Down syndrome, but this was alleviated after the amniocentesis test came back normal. My other concern was my age: Being an older mom, would I have the energy to cope? On March 8, 1997, a Shabbat, in the last month of my pregnancy, I stopped feeling any movement. We decided that I should go to the hospital right away. Once again, there was fetal distress, and I underwent an emergency cesarean section, under general anesthesia; and once again, no baby was laid on my chest.

My lovely first son was born two weeks early, but at a good weight. Nevertheless, the team rushed him to the neonatal intensive care unit, because one of his nostrils was closed. Once again I developed an infection after the birth, but this time I was also unable to walk. I was wheeled into the NICU, where I burst into tears, seeing my one-day-old munchkin lying in an incubator and surrounded by so many wires and needles that he was hardly visible. All around, newborns in the unit were dying. I just prayed that my son had the strength and gumption to stay alive.

Unbeknownst to me, my brother called in a rabbi who specialized in medical issues. He told my brother, "I'm so sorry, but this little baby is not going to make it." What a blessing that he was proved wrong! One week after his birth, on Friday night, our son came down with a staphylococcal infection. It was touch-and-go for a while, but God was with him and us. Usually on Friday nights, only less-experienced residents are on duty, but that evening, we were so fortunate that specialists were there who monitored his heart and kept a close eye on him. My husband was called to the hospital, because the baby was in real danger.

Two weeks later, I was released from the hospital, needing a wheelchair and a walker. The baby was still in the hospital, and while I tried to pump milk for him, I had very little. Finally, one month after he was born, he was released from the hospital and could have his *brit milah* (ritual circumcision). We named him Simcha Menachem Zev. Simcha means "joy." He was born in the Hebrew month of Adar, about which the Talmud (*Taanit* 29a) says, "*Mi'shenichnas Adar, marbim b'simchah*" (When Adar begins, joy increases). And indeed he is filled with joy and brings it to everyone with whom he comes into contact. His second and third names, Menachem Zev, were given in honor of my father-in-law.

I hired a woman, Efrat, to help me take care of Simcha, as I was totally out of it. I became deeply depressed after the birth, in good part because – as I had anticipated – I lost the ease of speech that I had enjoyed during the pregnancy. There seems to be something in the hormones of my impregnated body that allows for physically-easier speech. (In fact, my doctor tried to simulate pregnancy, but it did

not work: I guess there is nothing like the real thing.) In addition,
I literally could not move and was unable to do anything, let alone
take care of a baby, a toddler, and a nine-year-old. Soon Passover
was upon us, and we spent the holiday at a hotel in Tiberias. Every
day, I would go up to the roof and try to figure out where I could
jump from, and whether the distance was great enough to kill me. I
did this for eight days, but never found a suitable spot.

After we returned home, Israel's Independence Day came around
again. On this day, many people have a barbecue. My brother came
with another family to try to entice me to attend theirs: they thought
a little fresh air, delicious food, and fun company would restore me.
I had no desire to go out, however, and turned down their invitation,
staying with Simcha, who was fast asleep in his car seat. Then I took
one of Harvey's neckties and hung it from the rafter. I put my head
through it, but I just could not make myself kick the chair away. The
thought of my children or nieces and nephews walking through the
door and finding me hanging from the ceiling was just too horrifying.
I could not put them through such a trauma.

Nonetheless, suicidal thoughts did not leave me. Whenever I
had to take my children to the doctor, I would surreptitiously try to
obtain information about how many over-the-counter pain relievers
a person could safely take, and what would happen if one took too
many. The doctor told me that taking too much could destroy a
person's liver. My emotional pain was unbearable. I felt buried in
the deepest, darkest, blackest hole, which I could never crawl out
of. And really, I had no desire to, anyway, and thought I would not
be able to go on living.

I felt as if someone were holding my head underwater. I could
not see the light that maybe one day the depression would abate.

I could not feel the gratitude for all the blessings in my life that
I did have.

I could not fathom the fact that there were people out there who
loved me and would be devastated if I were gone.

I could not see beyond the darkness of that big black hole. It totally engulfed me, and I could not think straight. I felt that it would be better for myself – and for the world – if I were no longer around.

My mother-in-law bought an apartment on Agron Street and would stay in Israel from Rosh Hashanah through Pesach and then go back to Los Angeles. Knowing that she would be away for a few days, I drove my electric cart to her house and hid it in the bushes. I entered her apartment armed with about fifty tablets of acetaminophen. After I had swallowed them all, everything went fuzzy. Thank God, my mother-in-law returned home early and found me lying on the floor. She called an ambulance, and I was rushed to Jerusalem's Shaare Zedek Medical Center. There, they pumped my stomach. Various friends and relatives stayed with me, taking shifts throughout the night.

When I was moved into a private room, a guard was stationed outside my door around-the-clock. (This was the protocol for suicide patients, so they would not try it again.) I remember Orit coming to visit me and asking why there was a guard outside my door. I quickly changed the subject to distract her, rather than giving her a proper answer; she did not mention it again.

Harvey and my extended family were in total shock. They knew I was depressed and felt totally useless, but they had not realized the extent or intensity of my feelings, and what a life-threatening situation I was in.

I was totally unable to cope and would lie in bed all day, staring at the wall. When my mother learned what had happened, she and my sister Wendy came from the United States to try to help me. We visited a few psychiatrists, who told me I would need years of psychoanalysis. This was *not* what I wanted to hear: I needed immediate help.

I finally found a psychiatrist who suggested that I start taking antidepressant medication. First he gave me Prozac (fluoxetine), which was ineffective. He then tried Viepax (venlafaxine, also known as Effexor), which literally saved my life. Once the Viepax kicked in, I felt that I was on an even keel and could finally function again. I kept wondering, however, what had happened to that deep, dark, black hole. I was diagnosed with postpartum depression, a chemical imbalance which the Viepax remedied. Although I had not realized it at the time, I had also experienced postpartum depression with my first two children, although it had been less severe. Nor was it a well-known malady back then.

I could finally rejoin humanity and reestablished a better routine, despite still being cramped into our little apartment: Orit had one room; Harvey and I had the second room, and the two younger children were sleeping in the living room. We had had enough. We needed a house with a front yard and a backyard, like I was used to having in Los Angeles. My sister-in-law Marla and her family were living in Efrat, a community over the Green Line (in Judea and Samaria, or the West Bank), which then had about 6,400 residents. We decided to go and check it out. We found the perfect house there with three stories and a back yard. There was also an extra apartment downstairs, with its own separate entrance. We really liked it and felt it really suited our family's requirements, so we moved there in September 2001.

I needed to help my children get used to their new schools while I became acclimatized to a new community. Children are resilient, adapting quickly to changes, but it took me a little longer. I found the community very supportive on a personal level, but even today I feel that I do not quite fit in and never will. I am just too different because of my illness. There is a good deal of ignorance in the world about how to cope with and respond to people who are in some ways not the norm. Some people are even afraid that they will catch dystonia if they associate with me. Looking back, I think Nechama and Simcha sensed, even at a young age, that there was something different about me. This caused them to generally prefer their father, until they got older and started to bond with me.

I vividly remember Harvey going out one evening and two little toddlers standing at the door screaming and putting their arms out for him to pick them up and take them out with him rather than be left in the house alone with their mother, who was standing in the background. I cannot begin to describe how painful that was for me.

5 *Challenges and Opportunities*

Shouldering the Burden

> I was in a constant state of wrestling with the Divine.

One day, as I entered the house, my left arm shot up in the air and would not go down. I walked around with my arm in the air, which caused great pain. Somehow, I figured out that if I put a book under my armpit, my arm would stay down because it was holding the book. I searched through my bookshelves trying to find a book that would fit under my pit and that was also a good weight. Ironically, the perfect fit was the book *Wrestling with the Divine: A Jewish Response to Suffering* by Rabbi Shmuley Boteach. This book and I became inseparable. In any case, I was in a constant state of wrestling with the Divine, so why not wear my badge on my person?

Despite my creative solution, my shoulder became progressively more painful as the days continued. I was sent for an MRI, which showed that I had a very badly torn rotator cuff (in fact, there was hardly anything left of the cuff tissue), and I was riddled with arthritis. I spent most of my days in a steaming hot bath, where I was pain-free. After getting out of the bath, however, it would just be a matter of time before the pain returned, eventually again becoming so unbearable that I would get back into the bath. I also had to lie

44

down with my head raised up, which lifted my shoulder so it would not touch anything. I went to an orthopedic surgeon, who decided that I needed a shoulder replacement.

I went to another surgeon who was supposed to be experienced in such surgeries. He informed me that he did one such surgery every two months or so. That did not seem very experienced to me.

We then contacted the well-known medical advocate Rabbi Avraham Elimelech Firer, an expert in matching people afflicted by medical issues with the best doctor for them. He suggested an orthopedic surgeon in New York, Dr. Joseph D. Zuckerman. After contacting Dr. Zuckerman by email, we learned that he does at least ten shoulder replacements every day. Of course, we chose to work with him. I sent him all my records, and he scheduled my surgery for the following month.

At the same time, I was having pain in my upper thigh and lower back. A doctor on Dr. Zuckerman's team who specialized in this area happened to be working in Jerusalem at the time. After examining me, he concluded that I would need surgery for my thigh and lower back problems, as well. So I was scheduled for a two-for-one special.

My mother planned to come to New York to take care of me. Harvey was going to come with me for a week so we could see some Broadway shows and enjoy New York a little. We arrived at the New York airport and were picked up by the Tel Aviv car service company – an East Indian driver sporting a turban – which we had prearranged from Israel. We had planned on going straight to the Memorial Sloan Kettering Cancer Center to visit a friend, Shaindy Feuerstein, *z"l*, who was being treated for cancer. To save time, Harvey said the morning prayers in the car. Just as he was putting his tefillin away, the car crashed into a steel girder. We were not wearing seat belts – Harvey was thrown against the door handle and knocked unconscious.

An ambulance arrived. Harvey was so disoriented that he started wrestling with and punching the drivers. Finally, he was placed on a stretcher and put into the ambulance.

I needed to get into my suitcase to find my sisters' phone numbers so that they could be called. Because I was unable to talk clearly and had difficulty walking, the paramedics assumed I was injured also, so they strapped me onto a stretcher and put me in the ambulance, as well. One feels so vulnerable and helpless tied to a stretcher: people are talking to you from up above while you remain immobile down below.

We arrived at the nearest hospital, and Harvey was rushed into the emergency room. I released myself from my stretcher and went to find him. Unbeknownst to me, the emergency room nurses were looking all over for me.

I finally found him in a room attached to tubes and wires. The doctor said Harvey needed a CT scan. We waited, and after learning that everything was OK, he was discharged. By this time, my sisters had arrived at the hospital, so they drove us to the Affinia Dumont Hotel, where our mother was going to meet us.

Later that evening, Harvey went to my sister Wendy's house and was playing on the computer with her daughter Leigh when he passed out. Wendy called her doctor, and they met him in the emergency room of a different hospital. Harvey was unconscious and having seizures. He had a very bad concussion and some bleeding in the brain. He was admitted to the hospital unconscious and missed a whole Shabbat. I stayed in the hospital with him and am so grateful to the Bikur Cholim Committee (who come to visit the sick). They brought me kosher food, made Kiddush, and sang Shabbat songs, bringing with them the Shabbat spirit, which eased my fear as I waited to see what my husband's prognosis was. Thank God, eventually he had a complete recovery, but it was terrifying in those first days before we knew he would be all right.

A few days after the accident, it was time for me to have my surgery, so I left Harvey in the hospital in the care of my sisters while

I was in the hands of my mother. The shoulder replacement surgery lasted about two hours, and they also performed the back surgery.

The post-surgical recovery entailed intense pain, but I am blessed with a high pain tolerance. I did not take much medicine because it made me drowsy and knocked me out. I dislike the feeling of being out of control. The physical therapy started immediately while I was still in my hospital bed. I stayed in the hospital for three days and then had to wait another ten days until the staples could be removed. At that point I could fly home.

In the meantime, Harvey was still in the hospital, about to be discharged. The bleeding in his brain had stopped and the concussion had sorted itself out. He was put on medication for his seizures.

Finally, it was time to fly home and reunite with our children, who were frightened because they did not know the details of the accident. Fortunately, once we saw them, we explained everything and managed to put their minds at ease.

I was scheduled for six months of rigorous physical therapy. The surgery was on my left shoulder, and I am right-handed, so there was some consolation in that I could still do things. The physical therapy was very intense and sometimes painful, but it was a success: I regained full range of motion in my arm.

A year later, my shoulder began popping out of its socket. Each time this happened, I experienced excruciating pain. Harvey would drive me to the emergency room, where I would be placed under general anesthesia to put the shoulder back in place. After this happened three times, we decided it was time to call Dr. Zuckerman. He said I would have to return to New York for a reverse shoulder surgery. When a person's rotator cuff is torn, these muscles no longer function. The reverse shoulder replacement relies on the deltoid muscles instead of the rotator cuff to power and position the arm.

Back I went to New York, to go through the procedure all over again, with the same regime afterward. At one point during my second recovery, my mother was giving me a hug when she felt something hard in my back. I had forgotten that in my back surgery, which I had right after the first shoulder replacement, the doctor had inserted a bone-growth stimulator that needed to come out. So, after my shoulder replacement was done, I went back to the hospital to remove the stimulator.

I was initially given a local anesthetic, but during the procedure to remove the device, I started hitting the doctors and nurses, yelling and screaming. So they put me under general anesthesia. I was suffering from significant pain following that procedure, especially combined with the postoperative pain following my reverse shoulder replacement. Suffice it to say that I was not a happy camper. I managed to dull the pain with analgesics when I decided to take them. Then it was back to Israel for another six-month program of rigorous physical therapy. As we had no health insurance in the United States, all these procedures had to be paid for out of pocket. My parents generously and graciously took care of everything.

Shatnez and the Second Intifada

I had no idea what I was getting myself into.

In 2005, I attended a class given by a local rabbi, Rabbi Menachem Schrader, on the importance of not wearing *shatnez* – clothing made from a mixture of wool and linen. When it seems as if life is not going well, Jews are often told to check whether their mezuzot (parchment containing Bible verses, attached to the doorpost) are in proper condition, and or whether any of their clothing contains *shatnez*. Many believe that *shatnez* blocks prayers from being answered, perhaps leaving some of them stuck somewhere on the way to Heaven.

Rabbi Yaakov Gurvitz advises, "Find the *shatnez*, repent, and break the wall that blocks our connection to God." Things are never actually "wrong." God loves us, and He is all good, so we believe that everything He does is for the good. Everything that one thinks is "wrong" is a wake-up call specifically designed to help one grow and reach one's full spiritual, emotional, mental, and physical potential. We are just human and cannot possibly understand the way God works. As Rebbetzin Orit Esther Riter explains:

> Every time a person faces a difficult situation, he can create a great *kiddush Hashem* [glorification of God's name] by recognizing that God hasn't abandoned him, that God is closer to him now more than ever before. He knows precisely what He is doing. When we know that God is with us we receive a great deal of encouragement and the ability to overcome any challenge that comes our way.
>
> We need to know that God is closest to us during our most difficult moments. He comes at times of hardship and pain to be with us to encourage us and to tell us, "I wish it could be different now, but this is what you need. Do not worry. I am here to help you." Whenever we are in pain, God is right there with us also in pain.[1]

Rabbi Shrader realized that no one in our area was checking for *shatnez*. It was the height of the Second Intifada and was very dangerous because the local Arabs were constantly throwing rocks at Jewish cars. I wondered how careful we were being in the mitzvah of *shatnez* when there was a real risk of being shot while driving into Jerusalem. I thought to myself, *probably not very careful at all*, so I volunteered to be trained to check for *shatnez*. I had no idea what I was getting myself into.

Traditionally, this is is a job performed by a man. Because the rabbinic authority was ill, and due to other unforeseen circumstances,

---

1. Orit Esther Riter, dailydoseofemuna.com. Used by permission of Orit Esther Riter.

it took two years to obtain rabbinical permission for me to undergo the training to become a *shatnez* inspector. Rabbis Gurvitz and Schocket accepted me, and I began training with them sporadically. I learned a lot about identifying different fabrics by burning them and by looking in a microscope. It was fascinating.

One day, I walked into the lab and saw the most beautiful skirt I had ever seen: it was made from men's neckties. A seminary girl, whose mother had sewn it for her, had brought it in to be checked for *shatnez*. For weeks and weeks, I kept dreaming about the skirt, and finally I turned my vision into reality. Collecting neckties from whoever would give them to me, and buying some very inexpensively from thrift stores, I proceeded to make my own skirts. I tried to find the seminary girl, to see whether I could talk to her mother and ask her if it was okay to "steal" her idea, but I could not trace her. I checked with a patent lawyer who told me you cannot patent a design, so my guilt was assuaged. Finally, Rabbi Gurvitz told me very gently that, to check for *shatnez*, one needs to have a scientific mind, and that I had a creative mind. This was his kind way of telling me that I was not getting it. I was let go.

I realized that my intentions had not been pure to begin with. In the back of my mind, I had wanted the esteem that would come with being the only woman *shatnez* tester in Israel. Without pure intentions, things usually do not work out.

When Life Gives You Neckties

> From every experience, there is a lesson, even if it is learning what one should not do.

All was not lost, however, because I had learned a lot about fabric and had become inspired by that tie skirt. From every experience, there is a lesson, even if it is learning what one should not do. I ended up sewing two hundred tie skirts, each one unique. Some have appliques on them, or pieces from other clothes. Once I start something, I tend to get a little carried away.

At first, I made the skirts with the ties as they were. This used many ties, and the skirts tended to be heavy when picked up, although they felt light when worn. After making a few such skirts, I discovered that they could be lightened considerably by opening the ties and taking out the facing. To do this, I needed about sixteen ties for each skirt. I also designed a label stating, "Heavy in your arms, light on your body." I did not want potential customers to pick up the skirts and think they were too heavy, without trying them on and feeling how light and comfortable they are.

Looking at my email messages one day, I saw a notice for a show in Chicago: this was a huge crafts fair featuring the wares of many different sorts of people. I applied, just for the fun of it, and was accepted into a new division called Emerging Artists. There were ten of us, including people presenting jewelry, clothes, and woodworking. My mother and I decided to go on January 27, 2009. After finding someone to build us a booth, I set up a hundred tie skirts on the racks. My mother and I each wore one as well; we were ready to go. The only problem was that this fair occurred right at the time of the economic downturn, and people were reluctant to spend. There were many viewers and many comments such as, "Wow, this is amazing!" but, at $200 per skirt (What was I thinking!), I ended up selling only four.

The fair was also held on Shabbat. As I am not allowed to work on that day, I asked my rabbi what to do. He said I could hire non-Jews to sell for me on Shabbat, and the proceeds would go to them. I found a woman from the Dystonia Foundation office. She sold a few pieces of my handmade jewelry, which I had also brought along. So we took a big loss on that venture, having to buy tickets from Israel and Vancouver, and pay for the booth, accommodation, and food.

However, I was interviewed by ABC TV. The interview opened with the following introduction: "Some believe neckties are becoming a thing of the past, but many are being recycled into a new fashion statement for women. ABC reporter Karen Meyer joins us with a story of a designer with a disability who also specializes in necktie fashion." Meyer continued: "Cheri Tannenbaum cannot speak due to her dystonia. She traveled to Chicago all the way from Israel to showcase her unique designs."

Then Meyer showed the woman in charge of the crafts show saying, "Designs by Cheri was one of the exhibits selected to participate in the One of a Kind Show. Cheri was selected to participate because she was really appropriate for our Emerging Artist Program. Not only is her work so unique and just dynamic and truly one of a kind, she has pretty little experience doing shows and selling her work, so she's just a perfect fit."

Meyer continued: "Cheri's dystonia doesn't define her talent, but has created some limitations – like communication. Cheri uses her Palm Pilot to communicate. Her mom, Frances Belzberg, translates for her."

My mother then read what I had written with my Palm Pilot: "When you're impaired in communication and mobility – which are the ways of the world – it's hard to find something that makes an impact. My love and performance of art helps me to do this. It's the combination of adding other materials and other accoutrements to the basic tie skirt, not just using the ties as they are, which creates the effect I want." My mother added: "This child that I raised, that I lived with for all these years, I didn't know she had it in her." The woman from the show then continued: "I've seen ties used in different accessories, but not quite like her use of them. They are just really funky, and I think someone who is looking for a real fashion statement can definitely find them in her skirts."

It was a little comedy of errors. Ms. Meyer, the reporter, was deaf, so she signed and spoke; she was very hard to understand, however, so there were subtitles. Together with my not being able to talk, we made a great team.

The interview failed to drum up any business. Counting our losses, my mother and I went our different ways back to our respective homes.

My tie skirts are all unique and, with the elastic waistband, one size fits all. People have told me that each one is a museum piece. I have not given up on my dreams of selling my tie skirts. For now, I have stopped making skirts, except when I get an occasional new idea. I have given many away to friends and others, so long as they promise to wear them and become my walking advertisement.

I have bags and bags of ties and tie pieces, but this does not stop me from collecting more for the future. Sheindel Weinbach, who runs a thrift shop, receives many ties. Not knowing what else to do with them, she was just throwing them out. An acquaintance of mine who volunteers at the shop told her about my skirts. Sheindel was so happy not to have to throw them out. Every first of the month, I pick up a bag or two of ties that she has collected for me.

Indeed, I have a passion for second-hand clothes: I collect them. They hang in almost every room and closet in our house. I could change twenty times a day for two years and still not have to wear the same outfit twice. I call this my second illness, but psychologically, I have figured it out. First, no matter how bad I feel when I wake up in the morning – which is usually quite bad – I can at least wander into my many closets and choose something outlandish to make myself look interesting. I pride myself on my unique style. Wherever I go, I always receive compliments on my attire. Second, I consider my body a canvas: my clothes are my palette.

I am to this day an undiscovered artist. I make big, bombastic, funky, colorful necklaces out of beads. I make outrageous skirts out of men's neckties. I make hats out of fabric. I make patchwork skirts and dresses. I think these are all an expression of the real, true me under my illness.

It is not fame that I want, although there is nothing wrong with fame. It is not even the money that I want, although money would come in handy. It is just that I want to see all my beautiful creations out of the bags that are sitting on my shelves and in my drawers and off the clothing racks – instead, adorning women all over the world.

It is not for lack of trying that I have been unable to sell my things. I have not found my market of gutsy women who will wear my wild, outlandish fashions.

At craft fairs, people say, "Wow! These are amazing, but I could never wear them." I think maybe I am a little ahead of the time. So I guess I will just have to bide my time until everyone else catches up to me.

Harp Lessons

> Perhaps it came from reading the Psalms and learning about King David, who played the harp, and imagining that I was hearing his music in my head.

In 2007, I suddenly began to have a desire to learn the harp. I am not sure where this came from, because I was not musically inclined and had never touched an instrument in my life, except for a piano for two days. Perhaps it came from reading the Psalms and learning about King David, who played the harp, and imagining that I was hearing his music in my head.

My introduction to the instrument happened at a crafts fair in the Alon Shvut community center, where I was setting up my wares for sale. At the entrance to the center, a woman was playing a harp. I was completely mesmerized and forgot about my booth, leaving it unmanned. When she took a break, I passed her a note and discovered that her name was Shoshana Levy. When I asked her whether she gave lessons, she confirmed that she did. It was a match made in Heaven. I became her faithful student. Soon, I bought my own harp, as there was no point in taking lessons if I could not practice on my own instrument.

When my children were younger, adding this class to my repertoire would have been impossible, but now they needed me less. Happily, against the backdrop of so many dramas regarding my health and pursuits, my children continued to grow and develop.

6 Milestones

Orit's Bat Mitzvah and Growing Up

> Throughout Orit's work with Yossi, he kept telling her that his brother Shlomo was for her.

At age twelve, Orit became a bat mitzvah, a very exciting occasion. To prepare her, I took her shopping for clothes. Although I generally detest shopping, we had a special time together, and she was all set physically.

To prepare spiritually, she studied with a local woman about some of the commandments particular to women. For her party I wrote a speech, which I gave to my mother and sister to read for me in their own dramatic way. I wish I could share it with you now, but it was mislaid.

Orit went on to high school in Kiryat Arba, near Hebron, where she thrived. After high school, she did national service, a civilian alternative to military service that is popular among religious girls. In this framework, she could volunteer in one of several programs.

Her first choice was Shalva, the Israel Association for the Care and Inclusion of Persons with Disabilities. The organization, run by Kalman and Malki Samuels, provides respite care for children with special needs.

The Samuels' son Yossi had been born healthy and able-bodied, but at the age of eleven months, he received a contaminated DTaP vaccine that left him deaf, blind, and hyperactive. As he grew, however, they needed to find ways to communicate with him. They brought him to the United States, where a deaf therapist named Shoshana Weinstock taught them the technique of tactile signing – finger spelling in Hebrew directly into his hands. From that point, Yossi was on his way. Returning to Israel, the Samuels remembered the promise they had made to themselves that, if they found someone to help Yossi, they would find a way to help other children with special needs, and also their parents. Thus they established Shalva.

I had grown up with Kalman in Vancouver, so I suggested to Orit that she introduce herself to him and tell him that she is my daughter. He was happy to meet her, but informed her that he does not hire even volunteers based on personal connections – what Israelis call *protexia*. "You will need to go through the whole process, and if the powers that be feel that your qualifications and capabilities meet our needs, you will be chosen," he told her. She did, and she was. In her work, she learned the sign language necessary to communicate with Yossi, and they had a very close, special relationship. Every year, the organization has a fundraising dinner in New York. That year, Yossi attended the dinner, as did Orit, who spoke on behalf of the Israeli organization. When Yossi travels, he requires a man to accompany and assist him, so his brother Shlomo went, as well. Throughout Orit's work with Yossi, he kept telling her that his brother Shlomo was for her.

The rest is history.

Orit and Shlomo's Wedding

> It was very special to stand there, hugging her, before I handed her off to her husband.

Shlomo and Orit became engaged, and were married on July 12, 2005. It was an amazing, beautiful wedding at Neve Ilan, outside of Jerusalem. The only sad, difficult part for me was that I could not participate in the frenzied, whirling dancing around the beautiful, radiant bride. (Strangely, I can dance perfectly well in my mind, but to actually do it in the real world is impossible.) Orit did draw me into the circle, however. It was very special to stand there, hugging her, before I handed her off to her husband.

Orit and Shlomo have been blessed with beautiful children: Emunah, Betzalel, Eliora, Tehilla, and Natanel. Orit is a hydrotherapist who works in a pool with special needs children at Shalva. She is also very involved in the Efrat community and serves as a member of the city council. Shlomo is a lawyer and a very involved father. They live in the young couples' area of Efrat called the Zayit. It is a ten-second drive and a ten-minute walk to our house. I like to keep my children close if they are willing.

Nechama's Bat Mitzvah

> May you use all your wonderful traits to go in the path of God.

Now it was Nechama's turn to become a bat mitzvah. It was a little easier the second time around. We had an opportunity for some bonding time while we went shopping for clothes for the celebration.

Then, to prepare her spiritually, we took a course together at Matan (a girls' seminary) about the commandments particular to women. This allowed Nechama to explore what *avodat Hashem* (service of God) meant to her at that stage in her life. When I was young, most girls did little or nothing spiritual to mark their reaching the age of bat mitzvah. Now, however, with mothers and daughters learning side by side, the classes enhanced not only Nechama's understanding of the Torah and its commandments, but mine, as well.

We held Nechama's bat mitzvah celebration outdoors, at Genesis Land, a center offering food, workshops, camel rides, and more, on the way to the Dead Sea. It turned out to be a very windy day. Orit, as a married religious Jewish woman, covers her hair, usually wearing a hat or scarf. This was the first occasion on which she wore a wig, which the fierce winds almost blew off her head. Nechama delivered a beautiful speech about the Torah portion read in the synagogue that week, but, because of the wind, could not stop sniffing and snorting the whole time.

Unlike the speech I wrote for Orit's bat mitzvah party, I managed to save this one. Orit was my voice on that occasion, and I can still hear it in the wind. She opened with an introduction from herself:

> From the time of my bat mitzvah nine years ago, our mother prayed and prayed that she would be able to say these words herself, but alas, it was not to be. So she asked me, and I always do what my Ima [Mom] asks... Right?
>
> Ima, I hope I do you justice. Ima is just very glad that she's here, because Nechama had to approve of what she wore, and that meant no tie skirt!

Then Orit delivered the words I wrote for Nechama:

> Nechama, I think of you as my shy, cuddly daughter.
>
> We are very rarely not in some form of physical contact, with you either sitting on my lap after you have eaten dinner or at the Shabbat table.

Be it your feet in my mouth or in my nose or lying together in my bed chit-chatting, rough-housing, or cracking up, you are always so close. I am very grateful to you that, without anyone asking, you are always by my side whenever we walk, no matter where, with your arms in my arms or your arms around my waist.

This pains me that at times you feel the need to take care of me when you are still young enough to be taken care of. On the other hand, as someone pointed out to me, I'm grateful that you have the sensitivity to realize my needs and that you have taken it upon yourself to fulfill this mitzvah of *kibbud em,* honoring your mother, par excellence.

You have many wonderful character traits. You are sweet, sensitive, and caring. You are smart, joyful, intuitive, funny, and fun to be with. You are beautiful inside and outside. You are also an amazing athlete.

May you use all your wonderful traits to go in the path of God. May you be able to ascertain your divine potential and have the will to fulfill it. May God grant you every wish that He deems necessary for you to fulfill your spiritual, emotional, mental, and physical potential and to realize all the wonderful thjngs that you have so far demonstrated.

I love you very much.

Simcha's Bar Mitzvah

I have a lot to learn from him.

When it was Simcha's turn to reach the age of bar mitzvah, Harvey took him shopping for a suit. My little boy in a suit was a sight to be seen.

For the service, he learned the Torah portion and a few

commentaries on it, with my brother-in-law. My husband, in his own inimitable way, helped Simcha connect the Torah portion to the significance of the event.

We celebrated in the hall of the Aish Hatorah complex, in the Jewish Quarter of Jerusalem's Old City. We felt that this was a very spiritual location for celebrating a boy's reaching manhood, as the rooftop of the hall overlooks the Western Wall.

Once again, for reasons unbeknownst to me, God did not want me to give my speech to Simcha myself, so Orit graciously lent me her voice once again. She was nine months pregnant at the time, and felt very exposed standing in front of the crowd to deliver my speech.

These are my words:

Simcha, your parsha [weekly Torah reading] is from the book of Vayikra [Leviticus], the most different and esoteric of all the books in the Torah. It contains the detailed laws about the ritual and sacrifices in the Mishkan [Tabernacle] and later, in the Temple in Jerusalem. Your portion also covers the laws of *tumah* and *taharah* [purity and impurity].

It is very short on narrative. It lacks the story appeal that Genesis, Exodus, and Numbers have, but it does contain many commandments. So it is very strange that our sages say, "Let the holy, young, and still innocent children of Israel come to begin their education by studying the book of Leviticus."

What does ritual holiness have to do with knowledge and the real world? In today's world, where anything goes, and every type of human and social aberration is condoned, if not encouraged, there is no room for a discussion of purity of body and mind and holiness of behavior and soul. As a result, holiness is not a popular subject for discussion.

However, the rabbis of old, who lived in the classical Greco-Roman era, were well-aware of the importance of holiness and purity in civilized society.

All the stories of our people, of our forefathers and foremothers, the Exodus from Egypt and the giving of the Torah, will be of little avail in helping Israel survive if they are not grounded in a sense of holiness and purity, both national and personal.

We must reinforce this and make moral behavior the practical way to behave in a world that has lost this. I feel that the way to maintain holiness is to carry with you at all times the following verse from the Talmud (*Berachot* 28b): "Know before Whom you stand." If you are aware that you are standing in front of God always, how can your actions be anything but holy?

Now, Simcha, I'd like to enumerate your many character traits.

You are sweet, sensitive, caring, loving, fun, funny, smart, and capable. And very handsome. You are a giver to the nth degree. You would give the shirt off your back if someone asked for it. You are the first person to volunteer when something needs to get done. You anticipate other people's needs before they even realize they have a need. You fulfill the mitzvah of *kibbud em* [honoring your mother] par excellence. If you don't have your arm around me when we are walking, you are screaming to Nechama to grab Ima [Mom].

You also wear many hats in this family. If there is a problem with the computer, the speakers, tape recorder, or any other electronic device, call Simcha, Mr Fix It.

If someone lost something anywhere... call Simcha, Mr Finder.

If there is a speck of dirt somewhere... call Simcha, Mr. Cleaner.

If there is something that needs to be done... call Simcha, Mr. Organizer.

Now you are thirteen, and you have the biggest and most important hat to wear – that of accepting *ol malchut Shamayim* [the yoke of Heaven]. You are now responsible to do all the mitzvot. Now your challenge is to wake up every morning, invigorated and inspired to chase after every mitzvah, be it an "easy" one or a "hard" one, in the exact same manner, with renewed *kavanah* [intent] each time, with feelings of love and fear of Hashem, with *simchah* [joy] in your heart and *kedushah* [holiness] in your soul.

I DARE YOU!!!

Love, Ima

When Simcha is around, everyone is constantly asking him to do things. And he does. I, as his mother, feel that perhaps he is being taken advantage of. One day I asked him, "Don't you ever want to say no?" He said, "No, I don't, because I know that I can get things done quickly and perfectly. And before I go to sleep at night, I check off what I did that day." I then realized that he loves to do for others – this is his purpose and function in the world, his raison d'être. Since then I have only derived pleasure and satisfaction from watching him give. I have a lot to learn from him.

High School Years

My children were generally thriving.

Soon, Nechama started high school. Like Orit, she went to the girls' school in Kiryat Arba. It was a big change for me, because she was to sleep there three nights a week. I was happy that her needs for food, lodging, and intellectual stimulation were being taken care of, but it left a void in my heart and in my house. I also worried about her traveling back and forth when she came home. This was during the Second Intifada, and there were daily shootings and bombings. I would call her in the evenings and hear gunshots in the background.

I wrote the following letter for her and had it framed. She took it with her to her dorm room and displayed it on her shelf:

> May these next four years fly by as quickly, as smoothly, as easily, and as successfully as possible for you.
>
> May they be years when you discover your passion and get an inkling of what your purpose in life is.
>
> May the proximity and availability of the Me'arah [the Cave of the Patriarchs, the burial place of our foremothers and forefathers in Hebron] be a spiritually uplifting experience for you.
>
> May you have *kavanah* par excellence in your davening [prayers] and in your Torah learning.
>
> May you choose your friends wisely so they will aid you in your spiritual growth.

Following high school, Nechama – like Orit before her – volunteered for national service. She served up north, in the Golan Heights community of Chispin, where she was to oversee the Bnei Akiva youth group. At the time, this branch of the youth movement was essentially nonexistent, and her job was to make it operative. When she arrived for an initial interview, the interviewers must have chuckled to themselves, wondering how this quiet, shy, reserved girl was going to do the job, and sure that the youth would run circles around her. Nevertheless, she proved them wrong. In a loving, dignified, modest, and respectful way, she had the youth eating out of her hands and transformed the group into a thriving, viable unit.

Many girls undertake a second year of service in a new place, for a different experience and change of pace. However, Nechama loved Chispin and the youth group – and they also loved her, so much so that she decided to stay there for her second year, returning home one Shabbat per month. This was also an occasion for me to write to her, and I framed the following, which she took to her assigned apartment and displayed on her shelf:

In your shyness and quiet you are able to move mountains.

May this year of *sherut* [service] be amazing.

May this be a year of spiritual growth.

May this be a year of emotional growth.

May this be a year of intellectual growth.

May this be a year of communal growth.

May you be so strong in your Yiddishkeit that you are able to share it with others in an inspirational manner that will be accepted by all.

May you rise up to all your new obligations and responsibilities.

May you leave your mark in Chispin.

Then it was Simcha's time to start high school: Makor Chaim Yeshiva. Although it was only a short ten-minute drive from our house, he came home just once a week – on Tuesdays – and every other Shabbat. He also left a void in my heart and in my house. This is what I wrote to him to send him off on his new journey:

With your warmth, your smile, and your giving endlessly, you are able to become the center of wherever you find yourself.

When things don't work out the way you would have liked them to, you don't let yourself get down; you just pull yourself right back up and continue, believing that the next time it will work out and be even better.

You are a quintessential giver. You would give someone the shirt off your back. You anticipate others' needs before they realize themselves that they are in need.

Simcha attended a yeshiva in the old city of Jerusalem called Ateret Kohanim, after which he planned to go into the army in a combat unit (a mother's worst nightmare).

My children were generally thriving. Harvey and I were on top of things, offering direction, advice, and suggestions when necessary, combined with a lot of praise, encouragement, and attention.

Then more problems began attacking my body.

7 *Let My Right Hand Forget Its Skill*

Carpal Tunnel Syndrome

When I cannot do my art, I do not feel totally fulfilled.

It used to be that the most stressful part of my day was trying to figure out what to cook for dinner every night. I did not mind cooking, but I never had any ideas about what to prepare. Now, because of Google and myriad cooking sites, my problem has been solved.

Then, in September 2014, I began experiencing pain in my right hand, the one I used most. After a series of neuromuscular tests, I learned that I had carpal tunnel syndrome. I have no idea where this came from, because I did not consider myself a candidate for it: I was not an avid user of computers. Nonetheless, I soon found myself going into outpatient surgery under full anesthesia, with Dr. Michael Chernofsky, a fellow Efrat resident.

You know what I look forward to every time I have surgery? Getting wrapped up in a cozy, warm blanket taken out of a heated cupboard. The surgery room is always freezing, maybe to keep the surgeons on their toes. However, to keep the patient warm and comfortable, that heated blanket is necessary.

The surgery did not take long, and I was soon home again, although the surgery left me quite useless for about a month. When I don't have my usual schedule and have no reason to rise in the morning, I tend not to get up until quite late. Not having the use of my dominant hand for that amount of time also left me feeling very bored: I could not do the things I loved the most. I could read, watch movies, surf the internet, and so on, which did broaden my horizons; but when I cannot do my art, I do not feel totally fulfilled.

Furthermore, I could not cook, so I gave all my recipes to my helper, and she cooked them instead. I felt that she did a better job than I did, so we have continued in this vein for the days of the working week. I need to light the oven or the range, because *bishul akum* (cooking by a non-Jew) is not permitted in Torah-observant Jewish practice. However, I do my own cooking for Shabbat, because I want my love in the food for the holy Sabbath.

The carpal tunnel problem was eventually solved, and I returned to my old self with a pain-free hand.

Right Shoulder Replacement

> I am used to being independent and spontaneous, and need my freedom to just get up and drive away whenever I want to and to wherever I want to go.

When I had my left shoulder replacement, I knew that my right shoulder was also riddled with arthritis and had a torn rotator cuff, both resulting in additional pain. I wanted Dr. Zuckerman to take care of both shoulders simultaneously, but deferred to his advice against it, since it would completely incapacitate me during the recovery period. However, in November 2015, I started having more pain in my right shoulder. To eat, I had to use my left hand to bring my right hand to my mouth. It was rather unattractive. Seeing this when I visited her, my mother suggested that I eat with my left hand. I am not ambidextrous, but I tried her suggestion, and it worked. So there I was, a right-handed person eating with my left hand. I still do this – the only thing I can do successfully with my left hand.

More X-rays, CAT scans, and MRIs, and it was finally time to have my right shoulder replaced. A client of Harvey's was celebrating his son's bar mitzvah at the Western Wall. At some point, Harvey started talking to another man at the ceremony – the father of one of the bar mitzvah boy's friends. This man, Dr. Mark Loebenberg, was a surgeon who had worked on Dr. Zuckerman's team before moving to Israel. So we hired him to take care of my second shoulder.

Instead of the regular procedure, Dr. Loebenberg decided to do a reverse shoulder replacement immediately. The surgery was successful, and I went home after three days in the hospital. The entire process was so much easier than that first time in New York. I was in a sling for a month before starting six months of physical therapy, three times weekly, with a terrific physical therapist. I started to do my art again, but it was too soon: The pain returned, so I was asked to hold off for a little while longer.

I am used to being independent and spontaneous, and need my freedom to just get up and drive away whenever I want to and to wherever I want to go. This surgery left me useless and helpless, needing the assistance of others to fulfill my every need. Being the free spirit that I am, not being able to do for myself was very limiting and challenging, but it was a comfort to know that, unlike the dystonia, this situation would pass.

It did pass: after about six months, I was back to myself. I have had to adjust only two things. I still need to eat with my left hand. And to put a scarf on my head, make a pony tail, or do anything hair-related, I need to lie in bed and put my legs in the air and do various other body contortions so I can get my right arm up to the back of my head.

I live in a state of constant pain of varying intensity in one limb or another. It's not clear whether this is related to the dystonia or not; it may be, but this has not been medically proven. At any rate, if the pain is excruciating, I will take strong pills. If the pain is less intense, I use ibuprofen just to take the edge off it. A scalding hot bath – which I indulge in nightly – is the only total relief I get … until I get out … and then it's back again. If the pain is bearable, I try to relax, breathe, smile, and live.

Broken Elbow

> Suddenly, I saw myself falling, and I was on the floor in the most excruciating pain I have ever experienced.

It was May 2016. My bedroom door was closed because I was just waking up. After my morning washing ritual, I needed to get a shirt to wear. I went into my closet and reached for the top shelf. The door was in my way, so I closed it. Then I stood on a low plastic step stool, which I use daily. Suddenly, I saw myself falling, and I was on the floor in the most excruciating pain I have ever experienced.

I looked at my arm: my elbow was dislocated and probably broken (later confirmed). I could not move my upper body, but luckily, I was close enough to the door to give it a little kick. Although I tried to yell, the sound came out like a little meow.

My helper was downstairs, and there was no telling how long it would take her to finish cleaning down there and make her way upstairs. It took her about half an hour. She kept hearing these little meows and thought it was a cat outside. When she finally found me lying there, helpless, I asked her to please call an ambulance. She called Nechama, who was at the post office. Nechama repeatedly called Orit, who kept hanging up on her because she was in a class; eventually, however, she answered, and she and Shlomo came over. In the meantime, Nechama had called an ambulance.

My husband was out of town in New York, which was a blessing because it spared him the full trauma of my accident. Nonetheless, this did not prevent him from trying to help from afar.

The paramedics came and tried to move me, but I could not be touched, so they had to bring in others who could give me morphine. There must have been about ten men in my bedroom, trying to get me onto a stretcher and into the ambulance. Nechama heroically accompanied me in the ambulance, even though these situations tend to make her squeamish.

In the ambulance, they must have given me more morphine, because I thought that this must be what an LSD trip feels like. Everything was spinning. Objects and colors were coming at me. I was terrified. I ended up in the hands of my calm, capable son-in-law. We had to wait in the hallway for an X-ray for about forty-five minutes, with me writhing in pain. The X-ray confirmed that I had broken my elbow in three places – a very severe break.

Dr. Todd Zalut – a familiar face because he too lives in Efrat – put me under anesthesia to set the joint and put on a half cast to protect it. When I awoke, I was told that I would need surgery within a week. I waited another two hours to get all the necessary tests for the surgery. Finally, I was released so I could go home for Shabbat.

I was scheduled for surgery with some Russian doctor whom I had never heard of. Then my husband had an epiphany: he thought of asking my shoulder doctor whether he also performed surgery on elbows. Thank God, he did. So now I was very happy and confident to be in the care of someone with whom I was familiar. Surgery was scheduled for a week later.

The doctor came down to say hello for a second and then said he had to go figure out how to put the puzzle (my elbow) back together. It was a hard feat, but he managed. I was in the hospital overnight and then returned home. We set up a makeshift bedroom in the playroom downstairs. Harvey wanted to hire a nurse, but Nechama said she would stay on a mattress next to me. I did not need any help during the night, so she slept peacefully. Once again, my daughter was taking care of me, but this time she was not only my daughter – she was my daughter the bride. Nechama would be marrying Betzalel (Bitzi) Hazen in three weeks' time.

8 Moments of Joy

Nechama and Bitzi's Wedding

> Once again I was a bystander,
> able only to watch the frenzied,
> whirling dancing.

When Nechama was doing her national service in Chispin, at one point she had to work with boys. They were very rowdy, with raging hormones. She realized she needed a young man to help her. There is a yeshiva in Chispin, so she called the rabbi in charge and asked whether he could recommend someone to help her. He gave her the names of two people to call. The first one she called was unavailable. The second one she called was Bitzi, and he agreed to come and see whether he could be of service. They worked very closely together on various projects. This led to dating and eventually to an engagement.

Nechama had to find a dress for her wedding, but, because I was still recovering from the surgery, I was unable to accompany her. This hurt my soul very much: my last daughter to get married, and I could not even help her find a dress. She took a friend with her instead. I was feeling able enough to go with her to her first fitting and could not believe it, seeing her in her wedding dress. Now the problem was that I had made a beautiful (if I may say so myself) dress for

73

myself for her wedding, but was unsure whether the cast would be off my arm. If not, I would have to cut open the sleeve – which I really did not fancy doing. In the end, the cast was able to come off, and I wore my unique dress. Although I was in pain, I was able to walk my beautiful bride down the aisle. The wedding went off without a hitch, but I needed to have a little conversation with Hashem.

"Hashem, if You do not want to cure my walking and my balance after forty-five years, I have no choice but to accept this and to realize that You know exactly what You are doing. I am begging you to please do this one thing for me that would mean the world to me. Could You just cure me for six hours on this wedding night so that I can dance with my daughter, family, and friends?"

I waited and prayed, and waited some more, but it did not happen. I was disappointed: Once again I was a bystander, able only to watch the frenzied, whirling dancing.

Marriage Tips for Nechama and Bitzi

> Look within and envision the image of God in each other.

For Nechama and Bitzi, I wrote a blessing and some tips for a meaningful, healthy and happy marriage:

Let her and Bitzi build a *bayit ne'eman b'Yisrael* (a faithful home in Israel).

Let them have spiritual, emotional, mental, and physical intimacy. Let them be able to talk to each other. Let them have sympathy and empathy for each other. Let them be able to hear each other and let them be able to listen to each other. There will be bumps along the way, but through these bumps they will grow

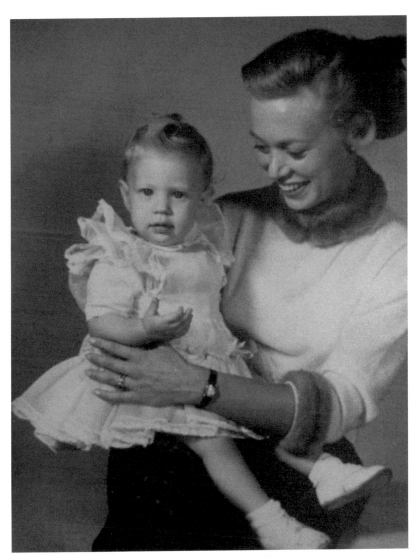

My mother and her firstborn child (me)

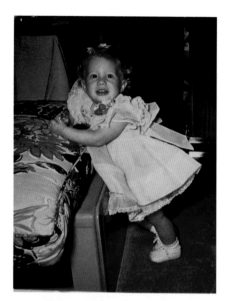

My two-year-old self

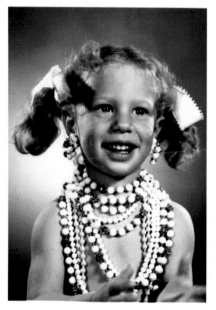

My destiny was preordained: my
mother's two brothers had a jewelry
store in Edmonton and used this
picture on their bags

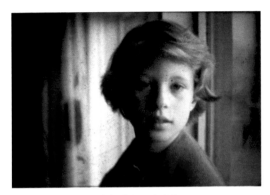

Me as a thoughtful older child

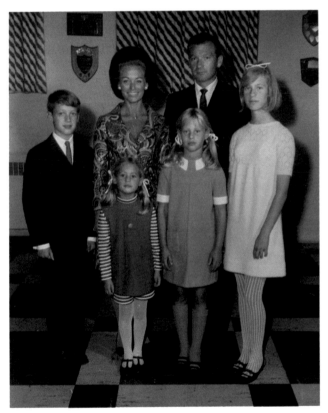

Clockwise from left: my brother Marc, my mother, my father, me, my sister Wendy, my sister Lisa, at my father's parents' house in Calgary, Pesach 1962

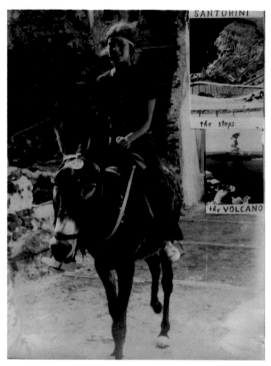

Me as a young teen, riding a donkey up the hill
of one of the Greek islands

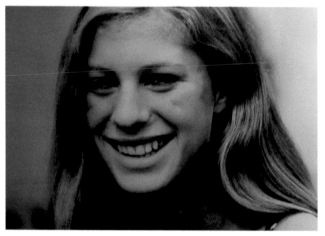

Me as a budding teenager, with my whole life in front of
me... or so I thought

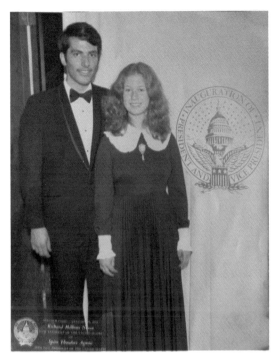

Harvey and me at President Nixon's inaugural
ball, January 1969

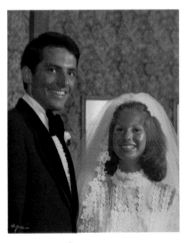

Harvey and me
at our wedding, 1974

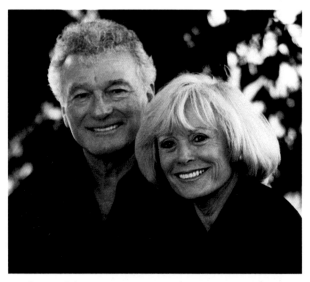

My beautiful parents
Samuel and Frances Belzberg, 1980

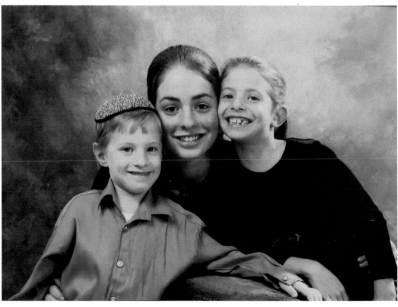

My children, *from left*: Simcha at 5¾, Orit at 17, Nechama at 7

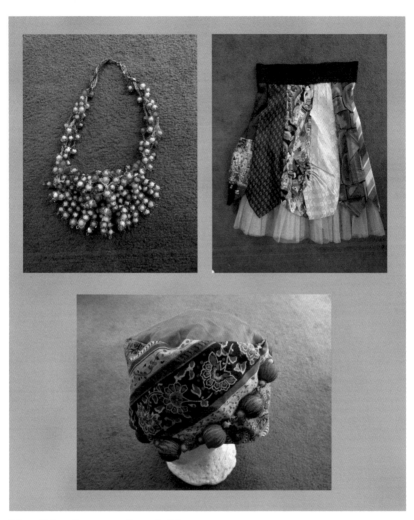

My wild and crazy, unique fashions

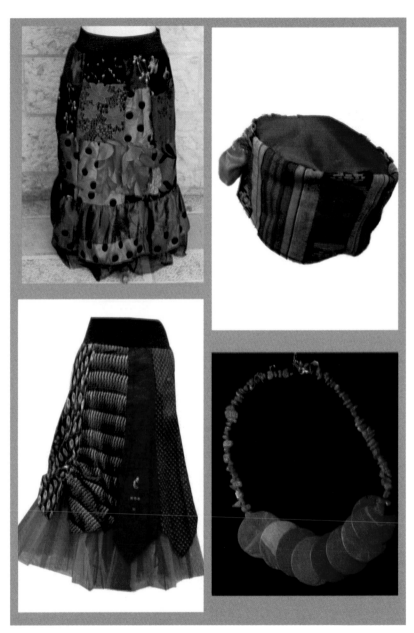

A few examples of my amazing creations

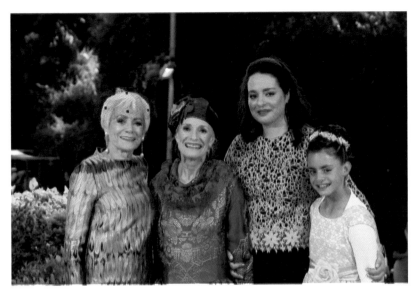

Four generations; *from left*: my mother, me, Orit, and Emunah, at Nechama's wedding, June 2016

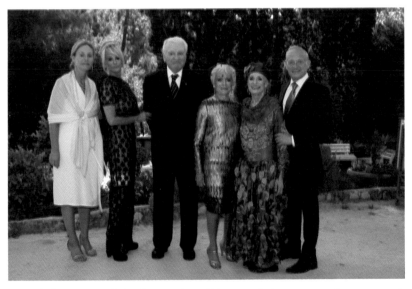

From left: my sister Wendy, my sister Lisa, my father, my mother, me, and my brother Marc, at Nechama's wedding, June 2016

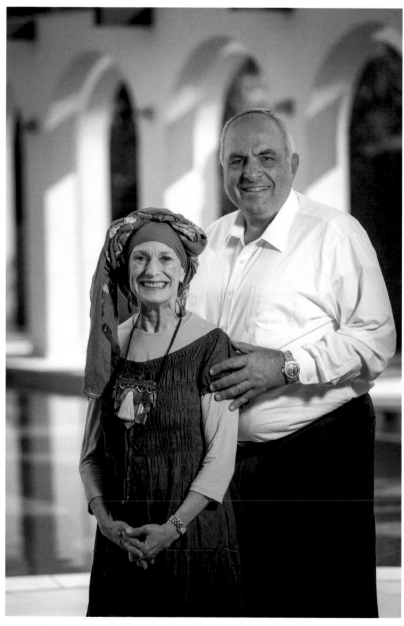

Me and my husband Harvey, at my mother's ninetieth birthday party in Caesarea, Israel, July 2018

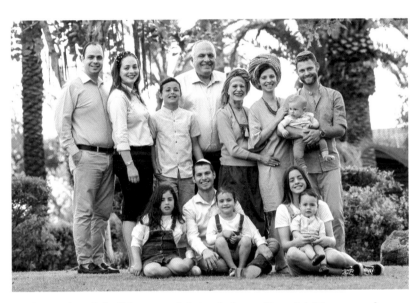

Back row, from left: Shlomo and Orit, their son Betzalel, Harvey and me, Nechama and her husband Bitzi with their son Roi
Front row, from left: Orit and Shlomo's daughter Eliora, my son Simcha, Orit and Shlomo's children Tehilla, Emunah, and Natanel

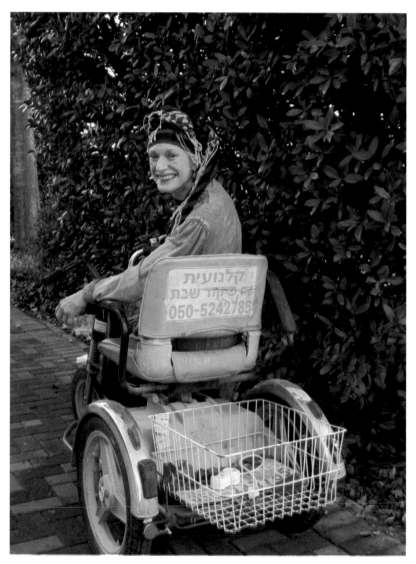

Me on my life-saving scooter, rigged by the Tzomet institution to run on indirect current so that it may be used on Shabbat, allowing me to socialize and not be stuck at home

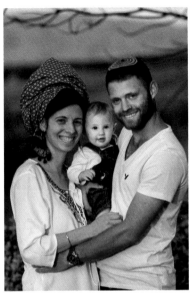

My daughter Nechama with her
husband Bitzi and their son Roi,
Pesach 2019

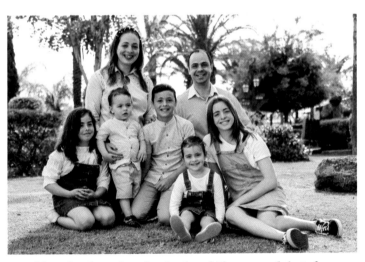

My eldest daughter Orit, her husband Shomo, and their five
children Emunah, 12; Betzalel, 10; Eliora, 8; Tehilla, 5; Natanel, 2,
Pesach 2019

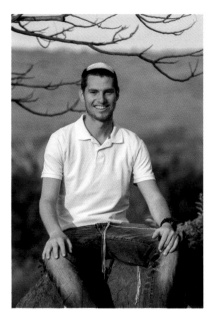

My son Simcha, Pesach 2019

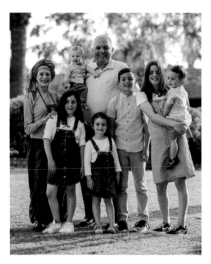

My husband Harvey and me
with our grandchildren Emunah,
Betzalel, Eliora, Tehilla, Natanel
(*in Emunah's arms*), and Roi (*in
Harvey's arms*), Pesach 2019

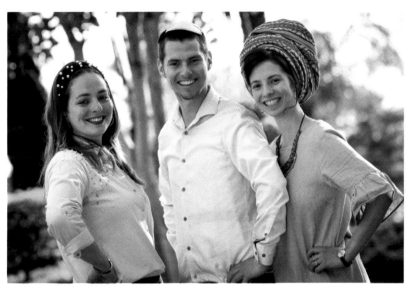

My three children, *from left*: Orit, Simcha, Nechama

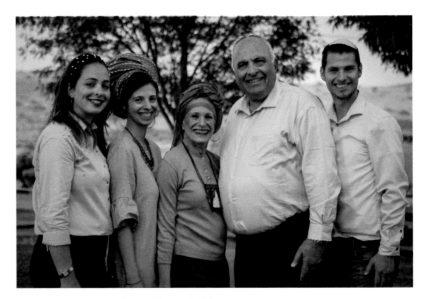

Me and Harvey with our three children, 2019

and become a stronger unit. Let them bring forth many healthy, beautiful *talmidei chachamim* and *talmidot chachamot* (male and female Torah scholars).

Look within and envision the image of God in each other. This will enable you to always talk and act toward each other with respect and dignity.

If one word of abuse leaves your partner's mouth or one action of abuse leaves your partner's body, you must stand up for yourself and declare, "This is unacceptable. This can and will never happen again."

Always keep the light of Torah and its lifestyle alive and exciting and inspire each other to grow ever higher in your worship of God.

Surround yourselves with people higher up the ladder to aid you in your growth.

Always try to challenge each other's minds.

Always try to have more soul talks than pass-the-salt conversations.

When one or both are angry, excuse yourselves until you calm down, then be sure to work out the issue until it is totally resolved, thereby promoting growth.

Always nurture your relationship. This is the most important thing in the world. Have a date night every week when you leave the house and go to one of your favorite places. At these times, children and any household issues are totally out of bounds. The purpose of these nights is to uncover more of each other's inner depths.

Always put your spouse first.

Always be thinking of what you can do throughout the day to let him or her know that you are thinking of each other and wanting to connect.

Never take each other for granted and always be grateful for what one or the other does for you.

Take advantage of the times when you are a *niddah* [prohibited from physical contact] to cultivate a deep and everlasting friendship.

Use the time when you are not a *niddah* to discover, experiment, and enjoy the pleasures of your bodies uniting.

May you be an inspiration to and an influence on all those you meet.

Love, Ima and Abba [Mom and Dad]

After the wedding, Nechama studied for a degree in informal education and worked with the youth in Efrat.

Bitzi worked himself up from a soldier in the army to a commander. As an officer, he came home every other Shabbat from Friday morning to Sunday morning. This is very hard on a marriage. Intellectually, they knew what they were signing up for, but I do not think they anticipated the emotional toll that this arrangement would take on them. They looked forward to Bitzi finishing his term of duty so they could resume "real life."

The builder of our house built an apartment downstairs. Nechama and Bitzi lived down there temporarily, while he was in the army. This way, Nechama as not alone all week: she could come upstairs whenever she wanted company. Their hearts are in Chispin (a two-hour drive from Efrat), where they hoped to move after his service.

9 Thoughts on Living Without

Being Unable to Speak Intelligibly for Forty Years

> I felt like I was wrapped in a cocoon of silence that was forced upon me, separating me from the world and deepening my isolation.

Communication, conversation, plain old talking – this is an art. Like any art, it must be constantly used, constantly practiced.

There is a different way to speak when you want to voice an opinion.

There is a different way to speak when you want your needs met.

There is a different way to speak when you want to help someone else get their needs met.

There is a different way to speak when you want someone to listen to you so you are truly heard and understood.

There is a different way to speak when you are angry.

There is a different way to speak when you are upset.

There is a different way to speak to have a deep, intimate soul talk.

Having been unable to speak intelligibly for forty years, I had lost the art of conversation. After being unable to talk for so long, I felt like I had nothing to say. I would be sitting in a room surrounded by people talking, and think to myself, "If I could speak, what would I have to say? Absolutely nothing." I felt that I was wrapped in a cocoon of silence that was forced upon me, separating me from the world and deepening my isolation. The silence became totally deafening, constantly reverberating loudly inside my head. I craved noise, action, and movement.

If you want a small, bitter taste of what it feels like not being able to speak to others, try the following experiment (and do not tell anyone in advance of your plan): The next time you meet with friends, do not say a word. Let it be as if your mouth is sealed. As the conversation flows from topic to topic, do not say a word. If you can manage to do this, you will gain a slight understanding of the constant emotional pain and seclusion of those with speech disorders.

I was afraid to get my speech back, and this could have held back my progress in regaining it – a self-reinforcing cycle. My entire speaking system – the diaphragm, lips, mouth, and vocal cords – was compromised. Uttering a syllable was exhausting. Furthermore, once I said something, often it was not understood, so I would have to say it again, probably not to be understood that time either. I wondered whether it was worth making the effort at all, but then I realized that if I did not even try, I would become a total recluse.

The Vorker Rebbe expounded on the idea expressed in chapter 1 of *Pirkei Avot* that nothing is better for a person than silence. Solitude, he said, is a balm for the soul, but only when one finds solitude *among others*. If a person is silent only because he is alone, he is not experiencing a spiritual triumph.

So I went out despite the challenges. Each time I left the house, I would have to think about exactly where I was going and exactly what I needed for the journey, anticipating every situation I might have to face. In the days of old-fashioned typewriters, I would type out notes to be handed to the people I would be meeting, stating what I needed, When I finally mustered up the courage to leave the house, I was constantly dodging – sometimes successfully and sometimes not so – people's insensitivity to me. Each (albeit innocent) attack damaged my psyche again and again.

My voice was totally without inflection or expression – a monotone – and my speech was completely unintelligible. To address these difficulties, I started taking speech therapy with Dr. Michael D'Sarro, a lovely, sweet, gentle, calm man with a lot of patience. He showed me what I needed to do and gave me numerous exercises to do at home. No matter how hard I tried, however, when my body did not cooperate – which was pretty much most of the time – I just could not get it all together and verbalize. It was beyond my control.

I tried another speech therapist, who suggested that I hold my nose when I spoke, to prevent the air from escaping and help make me a little more coherent. Doing this did help me become a little more intelligible, but everywhere I went, people asked me if I needed a tissue. In November 1978 I had pharyngeal flap surgery, which was supposed to have the same effect. The surgery worked... for about half a day.

Still, as with so many other failed treatments, I always felt it was worth a try. That is how desperate I was. I would try anything out there: conventional, alternative, even wacky. I felt that I needed to do anything and everything possible to try to help myself, even if much of that involved having things done to me, rather than my doing the work myself.

Of course I am not without weakness and self-doubt. I realized that I am always searching for that magic pill or magic person that will remove this burden and just cure me. In reality, I really have not done all that much to help myself. In some ways it is a little frightening to think of being without my dystonia, because then I would have to be a participating member of society. I have many fantasies about myself in that role, but so far I guess they are not strong enough to provide the impetus needed for self-healing. I say to myself, *I have always thought there was something called "mind over matter"; so why can I not conquer this with my mind?* On the other hand, I really do want to get well. Being in this condition is really frustrating and heartbreaking.

Now I have all the excuses in the world not to do anything; so what is the payoff of being ill? I cannot think of many. On the other hand, there are plenty of disadvantages, which include not being able to talk with ease – not being listened to, not being heard, not being able to make an impact – all of these being very discouraging, to say the least. Not being able to walk with ease, not being able to be a participating entity in society, being isolated, being depressed, having no energy.

The one redeeming result of illness is that everyone thinks I am so amazing, such an inspiration the way I fight day in and day out under these harsh conditions and never give up. Why, instead of feeling a tautness and weakness from the tip of my toes to the top of my head, can I not feel instead strength of conviction, the power of my mind and my will to just bounce back, and put this chapter of my life behind me? What is preventing me from healing myself, or at least being a participant in my own healing? God in His infiniteness feels that for some reason only He is privy to, I need this test for me and for the world. Until I have fulfilled its purpose, I will not be rid of it.

Whenever I went out into the world, I was armed with the trusty note that I had printed in Hebrew and English. It said, "Hi. My name is Cheri Tannenbaum. I have a neurological condition called dystonia, which affects my speech. I hold my nose when I talk because this helps me to talk a little better. (No, I do not need a tissue!) You need to listen to me very carefully to understand me. Please ask me to repeat myself over and over again until you do. I am not deaf or retarded."

Despite this note, people would just pretend with me. They would nod their heads yes, or say, "Uh-huh," even though I knew they had no clue what I had said. People would also whisper, gesture, or speak very loudly and enunciate every word very clearly and very s-l-o-w-l-y, as if I were deaf or retarded. I wanted nothing to do with these people, because their fraudulent or inappropriate reactions made me feel that they were not interested in me at all. I would tell my true friends, "I will repeat myself a thousand times over – whatever it takes – for you to understand me." That is what I did, and my real friends stuck by me.

Once Palm Pilot devices came into use, and I could type to people, I made it my mission in life to sensitize people with whom I came into contact about those who are different. I would type, "I hear you perfectly clearly, and I understand you fully. It is just hard for me to speak." By doing this, I hoped that the next time they met someone who was different, they would remember the encounter with me and apply my message by being tolerant and understanding of that person's differences, rather than cateogorizing each person in the same way. After all, each person's physical issue is different and needs a distinct reaction. This Palm Pilot was great, but what was I to do on Shabbat, when electrical devices are not allowed? I bought a lightwriter from England. It is a small, elegant, and powerful communication device for those needing voice output. It has a two-sided screen so a person can sit across from you and read what you are typing. It also has voice output. Tzomet (an institution that deals with halachah in different circumstances) adapted it so it works using grammas, which is an indirect current and thus permissible on Shabbat in a case of great need (and mine was a case of great need!).

Sometimes I would try to make a phone call and the recipient would hang up on me. I said to myself, *I am not going to let you get away with this*, so I would continue to call them until I ended up speaking to someone. They would apologize profusely for hanging up on me, saying they thought I was a prank caller. Perhaps the words Maureen Bogoroch-Ditkofsky in the former wellness newspaper *Confidence Bound* can help illuminate my situation:

Cheri has several degrees and is highly intelligent, yet because her affliction affects her speech, people who meet her at first make assumptions about her without delving deeper. They shout at her as if she is hearing impaired. They gesticulate assuming she cannot understand their words, or the language. They assume she is developmentally delayed. Do they see a capable, intelligent and highly educated woman? No, they do not.

They see only what their filters permit them to see. That doesn't make these people bad people. It just means that their lenses need adjustment or defogging. Cheri wants them to see her as a woman who has accomplished a great deal. She is a creative entrepreneur, a friend, a mother, a wife. Spiritual and grounded. This is how she wants to be seen. She does not want to present to others as only a woman who has a "condition."

Instead of risking exposing herself to false assumptions and insensitive responses, Cheri has discovered weapons of mass instruction. She uses a Palm Pilot to type messages to those who assume that she can neither hear nor understand the words they have spoken to her and the messages they are sending.

Instead of shrinking, she chooses to bloom with purpose, to sensitize those who assume that different means disqualified. She types them a message that she does understand clearly what they are saying but she has difficulty because of her illness to enunciate in a manner that would make her words understandable by them. Instead of absorbing false interpretations, she has empowered herself to change their view and possibly also their vision.

That does not mean that she is not frustrated by her disease or by the challenges she faces. That would be senseless and unrealistic. She wears what she describes as an "armor." In this, she means the support of family, an indomitable spirit, an unwavering faith, courage, creativity and a sense of humour.

She has acquired quite deliberately the right tools to cope and feel good about herself. She accepts her limitations to a certain extent but chooses not to let them defeat her. She stretches herself and achieves a lot. This fills her up, fuels her self-esteem.[1]

One incident that particularly sticks out clearly in my mind is the time I went to Hamashbir department store, looking for a wedding gift for a friend's son. Seeing a salesperson, I wrote to her that I wanted a pressure cooker. She responded, "Oh, you *miskenah* [unfortunate, pitiful woman]! This is what you want." Then she yelled across the room to another salesperson, in the proper department. "This *miskenah* wants a pressure cooker." The two of them then proceeded to yell back and forth, "Oy, this *miskenah*." This expanded into a chorus of salespeople, all yelling, "Oy, this *miskenah*!"

Finally, I had had enough of the whole store calling me an unfortunate, pitiful woman. I wrote to her I am not a *miskenah*. Then she looked at me for the first time and said, "I'm so sorry. You are right; you are not a *miskenah*." Not content with this admission, she then proceeded to shout to all the other salespeople, "She is not a *miskenah*!" and they all shouted back the same thing in return. There was a whole chorus of "She is not a *miskenah*" echoing around the whole store. Now I can look back and laugh; but then, I was so humiliated that I wanted to crawl under the cash register.

I am reminded of the following words:

> I have a visceral response to being pitied. Of all the things I ever wanted in life, what I wanted most was *not* to be pitied. Everything else was a bonus.[2]

I too am a stickler for not wanting to be pitied. I couldn't talk, yet

1. Maureen Bogoroch-Ditkofsky, "Oh Say, Can't You See?" *Confidence Bound*, March/April 2008. Used by permission of Maureen Bogoroch-Ditkofsky.
2. Lieba Rudolph, "How My Perceptions of G-d Have Evolved," TheJewishWoman.org, October 21, 2015, https://www.chabad.org/blogs/blog _cdo/aid/2739653/month/10/year/2015/jewish/Pondering-Jew.htm. Used by permission of Chabad.org.

everyone around me seemed to be talking so loudly. In my own head, the silence reverberated.

Whenever I would raise a finger to indicate that I wanted to say something, everyone would say, "Please be quiet! Cheri is going to try to say something!" Then everyone would be watching me, expectantly waiting for me to try to painfully eke out some sounds that might or might not be understood. This was a great purifier of my speech. I learned to consider very carefully whether something needed to be said: most things are not important enough for the monumental effort it would take to try to say them.

At the same time, I had to learn that when there was something truly important for me to say, I needed to be really tenacious and insist that people listen to me.

Not being able to talk bestowed a great advantage on me, as I developed the best listening ear. With pride, I loved it when my friends told me that they felt comfortable telling me their deepest, darkest secrets because they knew that I could not and would not tell a soul.

I am sure that my children were embarrassed by me, but they never said so outright. I always told them that when they brought friends over, they should explain my issues to them so that they would feel comfortable and not be afraid. This, my children agreed to do. Once, Nechama brought a friend home and forgot to tell her. The friend started screaming and crying hysterically, and phoned her mother to come and pick her up immediately. It was terrible for all of us. The children I met, including my nieces and nephews, would scream and cry, and run away as soon as they saw me. I would go home and look in the mirror. What I saw was not some kind of monster. I just did not see what they saw, but this is what I was up against.

Whenever the opportunity arose to send my children some-where – anywhere – with someone else, I always jumped at the chance and shooed them out the door. I felt that they were not getting enough stimulation in our home. In addition to my inability to talk, for some reason Harvey – who had the gift of gab outside the house – did not speak much at home.

And then, in August 2014 – as if all this was not burdensome enough – I started having crazy laughing attacks: I would laugh hysterically and uncontrollably, right from my gut. It felt exhilarating and liberating. I thought, "Maybe I should start my own laughing workshop." It's the current craze, ever since Norman Cousins dis-covered the healing power of laughter. Studies have actually shown that deep laughing has powerful physiological effects on the body, including lowering blood pressure, reducing stress hormone levels in the body, boosting the immune system, and so on.[3] A sense of humor also improves your emotional state, which in and of itself supports health.[4]

My laughter would come at any time: alone, with family mem-bers or groups of other people, and would last varying amounts of time. Laughter is usually catchy, but not with Harvey. He would ask me to leave the room till I was finished. There was so much tension in the house, you could cut it with a knife. My children were negatively affected by this, and it caused a dilemma, as they did not know whether to laugh with me or to be upset with me as their father was. Their reaction tended to vary according to the circumstances.

Finally, Harvey had had enough and took me to my neurologist, Dr. Avi Reches, who diagnosed me with a rare form of laughing

---

3. For more information on this, see Sondra Kornblatt, *A Better Brain at Any Age: The Holistic Way to Improve Your Memory, Reduce Stress, and Sharpen Your Wits* (San Francisco: Conari Press, 2009).

4. See Dr. Paul E. McGhee, "Emotion: The Key to the Mind's Influence on Health," in *Health, Healing, and the Amuse System: Humor as Survival Training* (Dubuque, IA: Kendall and Hunt, 1999), https://www.laughterremedy.com /articles.dir/humor.html#Anchor-Emotion; Lawrence Robinson, Melinda Smith, and Jeanne Segal, "Laughter Is the Best Medicine: The Health Benefits of Humor and Laughter," HelpGuide.org, October 2017, https://www.helpguide .org/articles/mental-health/laughter-is-the-best-medicine.htm.

epilepsy. Rare? So what else is new? After prescribing a medicine that disagreed with me, he tried another, and it had the worst side effect in the world: suddenly I COULD TALK. Yes, God works in very mysterious ways. Yes, there are miracles – they may just take a very long time to happen. At the end of the day, we always end up getting our just due. Never give up. Your situation can change in the blink of an eye, in the snap of a finger, or you may have to wait a while. Perhaps in the end, however, it is worth the wait.

The medication that Dr. Reches prescribed is an anti-seizure medication called Lamictal (lamotrigine). The doctors cannot explain its effect on me. There are no side effects, and – a little bit sadly – no more laughing attacks, either.

This miracle happened on my birthday, and it was the best birthday present I have ever received. Ironically, on the same day, I lost the charger for my Palm Pilot. I was intoxicated with words, and with the sound of my own voice. I was deeply grateful to Hashem for liberating me from a forty-year prison sentence. Can you not see what a totally different person I am when I can speak? I am fun, funny, and empowered. I have a personality. I have been given a whole new lease on life. I was so elated and invigorated that I did not know what to say first. I chatted with whomever was around, and when everyone had left, I chatted to myself. My son said to me in jest, "I wish I had a mute button." I had to make it clear to him that neither he nor anybody else is allowed to shut me up. I was silenced for forty years, and now I have a lot to make up for.

I could go into a restaurant and order my own food. I could walk into a store, ask for something, and actually get exactly what I had asked for. Everyone could finally understand what I was saying – not only a very select few. No matter how long it has been since I was first able to talk again, I remain in total awe of this event. I told God: "It would really be to Your benefit to continue to give me my speech, because I will be a better soldier of Yours." After my continual chatter, I remembered that I promised Hashem a few things when He gave me back my voice. I had said to Him, "I am not going to give you a bunch of idle promises that I cannot or will not keep; but here are three baby steps that I promised to do when You gifted me with speech once again."

1. So long as I enjoy the gift of speech from You, I will try my hardest not to listen to and or speak *lashon hara* (harmful speech, including gossip, slander, revealing private information, and basically any words that hurt another person).

    When I was unable to speak, I never spoke *lashon hara* because talking was so labored and effortful and took such constant concentration that I could not waste it on idle talk. In those years, I had to concentrate on every letter that I uttered. I had to scrounge around for words that did not require lip closure because this was particularily hard for me. Now, with the words rolling off my tongue, I have to make a concerted effort not to fall into harmful patterns. As Rebbetzin Tziporah Heller once wrote on Naaleh Torah Online, "Most of our sins are peripherally related to speech. Therefore, the key to control the *yetzer hara* [evil inclination] is to keep our mouths closed."

2. So long as You continue to bless me with the gift of speech, whenever I pray, I will say every word with my mouth and my eyes.

3. So long as I am still blessed with the gift of speech from You, I will try to do more *chesed* (kind deeds).

    The *chesed* that I started doing right now is picking up hitchhikers, because I can finally tell them where I am going.

    There are absolutely no words to describe how grateful I am to God for finally granting me the gift of speech. Now I am ready to have a reciprocal soul relationship with Him, after really doing nothing for Him for the last forty years.

Then I thought to myself, *How* chutzpadik *[impudent] is that?! After God's not really been on my radar all that much for the last forty years, He finally gives me back what I so desperately needed, what I so desperately wanted, and* now *I am ready to renew our bond?* On the other hand, I thought that perhaps God had been yearning to hear from me for forty years, and now it would bring Him great happiness for me to share my gift with Him.

Now I asked myself how one goes about having a relationship with God.

I asked my rabbi, Rabbi Baruch Taub. He told me, "There are four components," which he enumerated as follows:

1. **Count your blessings.** I do this constantly.
2. **Be grateful for what you have.** I am very grateful I am not envious or jealous of anyone's material acquisitions, nor do I covet anyone's possessions. I have everything I need and want, and much more besides. There is one thing I am envious of, which is totally allowed: I am envious of the Torah learning of other people and their children.

   I keep a gratitude journal: every night before I go to sleep, I write down the things that happened to me that I am grateful for, no matter how hard or humiliating my day was. Hopefully the good outweighs the bad, and this helps to change my perspective on life.

3. **Be in awe of Hashem's creations.** I am so much in awe that I will stop wherever I am – even in the middle of the highway (if there are cars behind me, I will pull over) – and in the middle of what I am doing to take a photograph of a stunning sunset, a unique cloud formation, a beautiful flower, rock, tree, or person.

   Whenever I go to a zoo, a safari, or anything else along those lines, I cannot help but see and feel Hashem:
   So many different species of wild animals
   So many different species of domestic animals
   So many different species of birds
   So many different species of reptiles
   So many different species of insects

So many different species of fish

Each with its own individualized markings and unique purpose to fulfill in this world.

4. **Talk to Hashem.** I talk constantly to Hashem throughout my
day, asking Him for help with all kinds of things. (For example,
"Please help me to thread my sewing machine needle." "Please
help me to open up my bottle of water.") Then I will thank Him
for helping me. I will also thank Him for not helping me to do
something. This lets me know that I did not need that particular
request at this time, thus obliging me to revamp my priorities.

I have understood this last one intellectually, but how do you bring
this down into your heart and really feel it on an emotional level?

To help me with this, I went to speak to Rabbi David Aaron, who,
I feel, understands God to the point it is possible to do so. He said:

> The greatest impediment to reaching G-d is that people have a
> particular idea of who God is from their childhood.... God is not
> this mean being in the sky needing us to conform to His wishes.
> God is not a separate being over there who is trying to oppress
> us by making us do His will.
>
> Your belief in God should bring you joy.
>
> Happiness is a state of mind.
>
> Addressing things of faith is a life journey. You must feel
> connectivity coming from a place of love.... The more I know
> myself, the more light of God comes out. To access the light of
> God, you need to be more true to yourself. To hear the voice of
> God is to understand what you know on your own, if you are
> in touch with yourself.... There is godly goodness that needs to
> come out through us.
>
> Love is the realization of shared oneness. Once you connect
> to this, you can't help but love others, which God also wants
> from us.... We are extensions of God. God is totally involved in
> our lives because we are a part of Him. God knows everything

about us, and identifies with us. We are one with God and with each other.

God has put in front of us life and death, and He says, "Choose life." ... Torah life is all about remembering and fostering the connection to God.

Mitzvot build our awareness that there is nothing but God, and I am connected to Him.... When you want what God wants, you have accessed divine will – the will that created the universe....

The mission is to choose goodness. You can transcend your nature and give presence to a godly nature in this world. Torah is a living testimony that God is one and we are all one with God....

What is perfect about us is that we are imperfect, with the ability to become a little more perfect each and every day.

Live your life for God's sake.... Trust God. God is also trusting us to make good choices....

Who you are is God's gift to you. Who you become is your gift to God.

All I can say is "Wow!" First, this is very difficult to understand, and it is even harder to internalize it and incorporate it into your life. It is a long, slow process. Hopefully, as you get nearer to the end, you will feel and bask in the loving embrace of God.

Always in the back of my mind is the fear that this medication's effectiveness will stop, and I will be rendered speechless again. I also cannot stop wondering how my children would have felt and how our relationships might have developed differently had I been able to speak when they were growing up. Suffice it to say that, in the end, I am very proud of how each one of them grew and developed into an amazing, incredible, special child (if I may say so myself).

It is what it is, however, or it was what it was. Because I was unable to talk for forty years, I have been rendered helpless. I have no idea how to take care of even the smallest thing. For anything that needed words (i.e., everything) I was dependent on my husband and children. I would call my children "my mitzvah secretaries," to make them feel that they were doing holy work. We all have our own lives, our own things to do, our own priorities, so it is understandable that my priorities were not necessarily their own. With no malice on their part, they took their sweet time doing the things I needed done. This was very hard for me – especially since my motto is "Do it now!" Now slowly, slowly – one step at a time – I am trying to use my speech to take my life back into my own hands.

My patience was tried once more; but then again, perhaps waiting for something is worth it.

Difficulty Walking for
Forty-Five Years … and Counting

> Whenever I want to walk out my door, I need to consider exactly where I am planning to go.

My walking and balance have been compromised for forty-five years and counting (for however long God wants me to go through this). When I walk, my right leg kicks my left ankle. It is exhausting and painful for me to walk any distance.

The only times that my wish for the gift of ease in walking has been greater than my wish for the gift of talking has been when I am traveling around and need to get to places. Whenever I want to walk out my door, I need to consider exactly where I am planning to go. What is the terrain like? Is it bumpy, rocky, or smooth? Is it uphill or downhill? Downhill is very hard for me, because I have absolutely no control, and I can just go rolling down the slope. Will I have to walk far, or can I either find parking or be delivered right to the door?

One of my famous lines is "It's just too far." For example, if I need to find a bathroom in a restaurant, and they tell me it is down the stairs and down the hall, well, "That's just too far," so I do not go. Because of my compromised mobility and balance, I have been hindered from doing many of the things I want to do and going to many of the places that I want to go to.

I say, "I cannot do these things." Truth be told, if I really pushed myself, I probably could, but I choose to avoid the pain, exhaustion, and fear over going and doing. For forty-five years, I have been in survival mode. On the one hand, I accepted my illness up to a point. On the other, I am very upset – to say the least – that this element of my illness is lasting so long. I need it to be cured yesterday. On the third hand, I have faith and trust that You will get us out of this mess. I just hope it will be before I am lying on my deathbed. It took You forty years to heed my plea for speech, and there are absolutely no words to tell You how grateful I am for this gift. I don't want to be greedy, but I need Your help very badly to cure my walking and my balance.

I must ask this of You because, one of these days, I am terribly afraid that I will suffer a very bad – if not fatal – accident. I cannot leave my husband wifeless. I cannot leave my children motherless. I want to be able to meet all of Orit and Shlomo's children and to see them financially secure and with appropriate and conducive living conditions. I would like to perhaps get to see one great-grandchild from Orit and Shlomo's oldest daughter. I want to meet all of Nechama and Bitzi's children and to see them financially secure with appropriate and conducive living conditions. I want to see Simcha out of the army safely with a *parnassah* (livelihood), a wife, and appropriate and conducive living conditions. I still have so much more beauty to bring into this world.

When my mind says *Go*, I either deny it and/or try to ignore the fact that my feet and my legs cannot simply go. I just want to get there. So, forging ahead as if I had no disability, I often go diving into something, knocking the air out of me, or I go crashing into something, cracking or breaking my rib, or even cracking my skull open. Come to think of it, it is a wonder that I am not brain damaged, considering the number of times I have hit my head on concrete, marble, or anything else in my vicinity. Sometimes, I do try hard to walk slowly, heel to toe, until I just become so discouraged, disgruntled, depressed, frustrated, upset, and angry that I let loose and get into trouble. Sometimes I will say to myself, *Okay, you will now walk from here to there very slowly, heel-toe, heel-toe*. Either I will do it, or I will not; or I will start to do it, become discouraged, and stop in the middle. I do have the capacity to control my walking and my balance, but it is just so mentally taxing. I must think of my troublesome feet twenty-four hours a day, seven days a week, when I would rather be thinking loftier thoughts.

I must ask God for His help around the clock. I know that this is part of His job description, but... I just need to realize that this is what Hashem wants of me right now – either to walk slowly or not to, and to end up getting hurt or not. This is my choice to make, or not. I know that You could heal me instantaneously, if You chose to. For the last twenty years, I have been giving You monthly deadlines as to when I want to be cured. Recently I have been giving You overnight deadlines. For the last forty-five years, You just keep saying no. I even asked You to cure me for six hours on the night of Nechama's wedding, so I would be able to dance with her, but, once again, You said no.

It can be very disheartening. Sometimes I feel like just giving up, but I will not allow myself to do this – because I need to keep asking, and I know that You need to keep being asked. So I will continue to ask, but I must tell You honestly that because of Your bad track record with me, I can no longer ask with true *bitachon* (trust) and true *emunah* (faith) that it will occur. (Maybe if I could, I would experience a miracle).

So it is one of my goals to be able to ask You for a cure whole-heartedly with full *emunah*. More often than not, I think this test is bringing out the worst in me, and I say, "Hashem, enough is enough, already. Fory-five years is a long time to cause a person to suffer. Our sages say that God never gives a person something he or she cannot handle. If, as we believe, You are also suffering with me, have You not also had enough? Would You not want to take one of Your suffering burdens – mine – off Your shoulders?

Sometimes I feel like saying, "If You cure me right this very second, I will never ask You for anything else for the rest of my life." And then I realize how foolhardy that would be. I am sure that, down the line, I will need something for myself or one of my children or grandchildren. The fact that I am saying this must make You realize how totally desperate I am for a cure for my walking and balance. So, once again as I say every night, I am begging You with all my heart, with all my soul, and with all my guts, please cure my walking and my balance by the time I have finished washing my hands in the morning.

I know that God has blessed me with so much, but when I have a test (my walking and balance difficulties) in my face 24–7, sometimes it is hard to see the blessings.

I so much want to connect to You, but you are making it very hard for me – even though I will never give up trying. If I cannot do this, then what is the point? Our purpose in life is to connect with You and bring down Your godly light into the world. Our sages tell us that those whom God tests a lot are very dear and loved by Him. I feel just the opposite – very unloved and picked-upon. I know that it does not work this way that if You do this for me, I will do that for You, or vice versa. If I am going to call myself an Orthodox Jewess, then I must walk the walk and talk the talk. Our sages tell us if you are not doing something with the right intention, just keep doing it and eventually you will. In other words, "Fake it till you make it." Then you just need to pray until God finds you worthy, or it becomes the right time to get what you need or want. However, it may never be the right time, because God may feel that it is not in your best interest to have it, even though you think it is. God always wins.

For the life of me, I do not understand why You think it is not in my best interest to be able to walk properly and to have good balance. I cannot fathom why God, a heavenly loving Father, would want to deliberately (so it seems to me in my finiteness) hurt me, His child.

I am petrified of crowds, because if someone just brushes past me, I will land on the floor – my second home, which knows every one of my body parts intimately – and then I may get trampled on. (It may not seem funny to some, but my sense of humor is what keeps me going.) In which case, I would need to go to the Efrat Emergency Medical Center, my third home, where I go to get stitched or glued up, and where I am on a first-name basis with all the paramedics and doctors: "So, Cheri, what happened this time?" I prefer to go there on Friday or Saturday night, because then it is free; but, like so many things in life, it does not always work out that way. My fourth home is any one of the emergency rooms in hospitals around the country, where I go for broken bones to be set.

Granted, part of my falling is my fault: when I want to go some-where, I often deny that my feet and legs do not cooperate. So I take off and end up in my second home.

At other times, I fall for no reason whatsoever.

So I have missed celebrations for soldiers at the Western Wall.

I have missed celebrations in Hebron during Sukkot.

I have missed going to the Western Wall on Shavuot morning.

And this is just the beginning of the list.

When I walk down the street, people are always staring.

They pass me and then stop in their tracks and turn around to continue to stare at me. A friend of a friend of mine who has cerebral palsy says she considers the starers her "fans." I like that, so I am going to adopt that attitude also.

Machon Tzomet, an institution that helps people solve various problems within the framework of the religious law, and Uri Dassburg, z"l, introduced me to a Kalnoit, a motorized vehicle that I could ride around in. It also has a Shabbat box, allowing me to use it on Shabbat by utilizing an indirect current. I could never walk my children around the block or take them to the park in a conventional baby stroller, but I could take them around in my motorized scooter. When they were young, I had car seats installed in it, and when they got older, these were exchanged for seat belts.

People always stared at us, and my children would ask why, as it made them feel uncomfortable. I told them it was because they were jealous, and they wished they could ride on the Kalnoit. This made them feel good about the whole experience.

It was not long before they decided to play a game, and started staring back. Seeing the starers become flustered, embarrassed, and self-conscious was fun for my children. I hoped this would teach the starers what it feels like to be stared at, and that they would refrain from doing so in the future. There is an important lesson here.

Now I can look back and laugh at what I call three "chair or scooter stories."

In the first story, I was in a Torah class at the Great Synagogue in Jerusalem, and I left my motorized chair outside. When I came out of the class, the road was blocked off, and there were lots of policemen swarming on the street and sidewalk. I sat down on my motorized chair, and one of the policemen asked if it belonged to me. I told him it did. He then explained to me that I had arrived just in time, because the police feared that my chair was a *chafetz chashud* (a suspicious object) and were just about to blow it up, which is their standard operating procedure in such cases. Calamity averted!

In the second instance, I was at the old Hamashbir department store riding around. A passerby told me that I had a flat tire. I called Amit, the man who fixes my chair, and he said he would come and help me; but he did not know exactly when. I really did not have time to wait around, but neither did I want to just leave it there, because it might be mistaken again for a suspicious object. Then I spotted three policemen. One of them was wearing a *kippah* (yarmulke), so I decided to approach him. I asked him whether he would be staying in the area for a while; if so, could he please watch my chair. He answered that he was leaving shortly, but added, "You see that man who is selling clothes? He's here all day. I'll go ask him if he can watch it for you." The policeman said to the vendor, "This *miskenah* needs your help." I bristled at being called *miskenah* again. The policeman explained that I needed him to watch over my chair, and the vendor agreed. I thanked the policeman and told him (this happened when I could talk, and I felt so good saying this with my own words), "I am not a *miskenah*." He denied saying it. I insisted, saying, "You did say it, and don't you ever call anyone a *miskenah*." He apologized profusely. So here, my chair served an educational purpose.

My third story takes place on a Shabbat, when I was riding my chair back from the Western Wall. There was a lot of construction going on, so the road was cordoned off. I thought that I would be able to get through, but I only made it part of the way before getting stuck at the part where a lot of Arabs congregate, which made me feel a bit nervous. I could neither go forward nor back. Suddenly, about ten black-hatted yeshiva boys surrounded me and began discussing whether the chair was *muktzah* (something one is forbidden to touch on Shabbat). For about fifteen minutes, they continued discussing the detailed laws of *muktzah*. In the end, they decided it was *muktzah*, so they walked away, leaving me stuck there. An Arab man was sitting across the way, watching the whole scene. When the yeshiva boys walked off, he came over and simply lifted my chair for me, and off I went. I just kept on thinking to myself what a total *chillul Hashem* (desecration of God's name) that was for an Arab to witness "righteous" Jews leaving one of their own stuck. This story truly has so many lessons for us all, including about how truly to serve God, and about not prejudging others.

While my chair is a great help, I just want to feel the Land of Israel under my feet. I want to be able to go hiking, camping, and exploring. I want to be able to go swimming, horseback riding, bicycle riding, dancing, running, jogging, walking, and so much more before I grow too old. I do all these things in my mind, but this is no longer good enough for me. I need to actualize it. Most importantly, however, I want to be able to dance at Simcha's wedding, since I was unable to at Orit's and Nechama's weddings. You have to unlock my shackles and set me free. You have to unlock my shackles and let me fly.

When Nechama was doing her national service, we went to visit her for a Shabbat. Everyone decided to visit a local spring. For a change, I did not want to stay behind, as I usually do. Instead, I decided to be a little adventurous. First, however, I asked Nechama whether it was difficult to reach the spring. She said that it was very easy. Well, her easy and my easy are worlds apart. We reached a big, daunting decline where I had to hold on to her for dear life. Then there were huge boulders that I had to climb over. Finally, we got to the spring, and it was really beautiful, nestled in the forest with the sun shining through the trees. I dangled my feet in the freezing cold water, thinking about how much beauty I miss because of my limited mobility, but deeply grateful for these lovely moments.

Whenever I am walking with my children, one of them is always holding me or they are yelling to each other to "get Ima." I find myself regressing to a handicapped person. Although I feel grateful to them for recognizing my need for help, I abhor it at the same time.

Had I been given the chance to say *no* to this disorder, of course I would have. But the experiences I have had and the people I have met are unique unto themselves. I've seen the human

condition up close and it has been compelling. Without dystonia, I wouldn't have the same perspective of life. Whether that
perspective would be better or worse I'll never know for sure.[5]

Oh, to be able to walk again normally and to have proper balance!
When You decide it is my time to be gifted with proper walking and
proper balance, I will be able to run after a mitzvah without fear of
falling. I will give away my Shabbat chair anonymously to someone
who needs it but cannot afford it. I will be able to take a walk, a jog,
or a run with my husband, my children, and my grandchildren.

I will be able to take my grandchildren places alone. Now, I do
not feel that I can keep them safe, because I have to focus so much
on where and how I am walking, and on trying not to fall. I do not
want them to have to be responsible for picking their grandmother
up from the floor. There are some things I would like to pass on from
one generation to the next, but this is not one of them.

I will do some kind of *chesed*. I am thinking along the lines of taking the latest shift once a week at the *pinah chamah* (literally "warm
corner"), a hut-type structure named for a man who was killed in a
terrorist attack, which offers a warm, friendly, cozy haven for soldiers
to come rest their weary bones and take some refreshment.

I have no idea what I am supposed to learn from the fact of my
constant falling and getting hurt. If I could just discover what I am
supposed to do with this, then I would be able to handle it with joy.
I would be able to work with it, and with You. I know, however, that
it is really not Your nature to give direct glimpses, so I will just have
to open my eyes and see where that understanding is hidden.

No one knows the reasons why Hashem does these things – but
sometimes Hashem gives us challenges and difficulties and we
wonder why would Hashem be doing this to us? The answer is

---

5. Brenda Currey Lewis, *A Twisted Fate: My Life with Dystonia* (Victoria, BC:
FriesenPress, 2013). Used by permission of Brenda Currey Lewis.

perhaps that Hashem has big things planned. The time will come. The time will be right. We can never give up hope. We have to hold on to that faith and tremendous *yeshuos* [salvations] will be on their way.[6]

I am hoping that one day – sooner rather than later – You will finally say yes to my desire to walk.

---

6. Rabbi Yechiel Spero, *Inspiration Daily*, Yeshiva Ateres Shimon. Used by permission of Rabbi Yechiel Spero.

10 *What I Have Learned*

Patience

> I have learned not to take anything for granted, because in a split second it can be taken away.

I have most certainly learned patience.

Patience waiting for the meds to kick in.

Patience waiting for people to understand my words.

Patience waiting for my grandchildren to start loving me.

Patience waiting for people to discover the real me under my illness.

Patience waiting for the medical world to unravel my mystery.

Patience for people's issues in general.

I have learned not to take anything for granted, because in a split second it can be taken away. Most of us do not appreciate what we have until it's gone.

I have learned what it means to be different, and the humiliation and stigma that go along with that.

I have felt pain, anger, frustration, and humiliation.

I have learned that I have strengths that I never knew I had.

I have learned that I have a fighter's spirit.

I have learned that I have courage, which is not the absence of pain, but the ability to move forward in the face of pain.

I have learned that I have a heightened sense of humor.

I have learned that I have an amazingly good listening ear.

It is said that silence is golden.

The fence to wisdom is silence. When a person is silent, he is not busy expressing himself, and this leaves room to hear things that come from beyond us. When we are silent, we are making room for another person. You can't listen while you are talking, but you can listen when you are silent. The power of silence is the ability to give another person their space. At every moment, we are making a choice of taking space or making space. When we are silent, we are making space. It is important to both take space and/or make space, depending on every circumstance.[1]

M.L. Cramer wrote in *Facing Adversity with Faith* that illness heightens our capacity for introspection, bringing in its wake humility, true friendship, creativity, and a deeper spiritual connection, and that it allows us to transcend the triviality that can so often characterize stereotypical health.

I have learned that it is important to give to others, for no reason other than transcending one's own self-absorption. There are others in more dire straits than you, not that I always find that comforting, because God has given each person the test he or she needs to reach their own potential. Comforting or not, always try whenever possible to lend your helping hand to another human being. Performing a mitzvah and a kindness not only gives the recipient a gift, but it also makes you feel good about yourself, enhancing your self-esteem and overall well-being.[2]

1. Rabbi Aryeh Weinstein, "Why It's Better to Be Quiet," Chabad.org, https://www.chabad.org/multimedia/media_cdo/aid/3101546/jewish/Why-Its-Better-to-Be-Quiet.htm.

2. See Eliana Cline, "5 Powerful Lessons about Giving," Aish.com, June 27, 2015, https://www.aish.com/sp/pg/5-Powerful-Lessons-about-Giving.html.

If I had had a choice, I would have preferred to learn these lessons under healthy circumstances, but I probably would not have. So, God, I am grateful to You for having graced me with these insights.

As Aharon Margalit, paralyzed by polio as a child, wrote:

> This is essentially our mission in this world: to transform our pain and suffering into applicable lessons; to collect the insights gained from the process of breakdown and survival and by means of them, to forge a path. In life, that means accepting, understanding, consideration and tolerance. Mainly being full of determination and faith that the path was meant not only for those who walk without difficulty.[3]

How I Carry On

I consciously and deliberately choose life.

Communication and mobility are the way of the world, and when one is affected in both these areas, life is a constant struggle. You may be asking yourself, as I frequently do:

What keeps this woman going?

What keeps this woman fighting?

What helps this woman haul herself out of bed every morning to face these seemingly unsurmountable challenges?

It would be so much easier for me to just crawl into bed, pull the covers over my head and never get up. From the first day of my illness to this very day, I wake up each morning, say Modeh Ani

---

3. Moshe Gutman, *As Long as I Live: The Life Story of Aharon Margalit*, translated from the Hebrew by Sharon Gelbach (Jerusalem: Feldheim, 2012).

(the prayer said upon awakening in the morning), push myself out
of bed, and consciously and deliberately choose life.

> I have set before you life and death, the blessing and the curse.
> You shall choose life so that you and your descendants shall
> live.[4]

Happiness is a choice.

I must take life every second as it comes. I know that my day
will be a constant struggle and full of humiliation. I try to surround myself with positive, supportive people. I take help from
others when I need it. (I always say, "I'm not helpless. I just need
some help.") I try to give to someone else, to transcend my own
self-absorption. I hear the call of God: "See how I am helping you
to bring out your greatness so that you can be an inspiration to
others." I hear the call of my husband, loving me and rooting for me,
and saying, "I still need a life partner despite your disability." I hear
the call of Orit, Nechama, and Simcha loving me and rooting for
me, and each saying, "I still need you." I hear the cry of the people
I know loving me and rooting for me and saying, "We all still need
you." I hear my creative spirit calling me and saying, "There is still
more beauty that needs to be put into this world."

After I made aliyah to Israel, a *Jerusalem Post* reporter wrote about
me, "Armed with intelligence, creativity, a sense of humor and an
indomitable spirit, there are no challenges Cheri has not been able
to meet head-on and prevail."[5] I try to make sure that continues to
be true.

I ask God to give me the strength to cope.

I live life one second at a time.

I once heard a rabbi say that our suffering is precious to God.

---

4. Deuteronomy 30:19.
5. Ruth Beloff, "Arrivals: Cheri Tannenbaum – From Edmonton to Efrat,"
Jerusalem Post, June 19, 2008.

WHAT I HAVE LEARNED

When we persevere in fighting for what is meaningful to us, in seeking God in our daily lives despite heavy obstacles, God feels about us the way we do when we see our brand-new toddlers fall down as they try to take a step and then get right back up again and keep chugging along.

Whatever situation you find yourself in, at any time or in any place, if you are in the moment, doing what is called for wholeheartedly, you are fulfilling your purpose at that time. Another way to fulfill your purpose is to discover who you are. You need to discover your strengths, your talents, and your passions and run with them. I have been blessed to have found my passion – my art.

I take art classes daily: beading, weaving, metal jewelry, collage, sewing, and papier-mâché. All my lessons are private, because they need to suit my body's rhythms. My circadian clock is totally backward: I go to sleep at 3 a.m. and sleep very fitfully until I must get up for my first class. Every time I turn over – which is frequent – I wake up. I also wake up a lot from pain. I end up feeling more tired in the morning than I was before I went to bed. But I do get up every day and launch myself once again into my art. I will run with it, wherever it takes me, and try to bring more exquisiteness into this beautiful world.

Hitbodedut, My Private Prayer

> I believe we should always be active and creative participants in prayer and all aspects of life.

Prayer has a purpose in its own right, which directly affects the existence of the world and draws the person who is praying closer to God. Rabbi Shneur Zalman of Liadi stressed that prayer needs to be continuous, like a thread. The slightest fray, and the thread unravels and tears.

I am unable to pray from a prayer book. The words in the prayer book do not speak to me – my eyes just roll off them. I know that standardized prayer is very important: it covers everything needed to be said in a systematic fashion and unifies the Jewish people by ensuring that everyone says the same thing. However, it just doesn't work for me. I know if everyone felt this way, there would be utter chaos, but I must do what is best for me.

Praying the same thing three times a day from the time you can read until age 120 can become robotic and even deadening. I do not believe we should ever be robotic, but always active and creative participants in prayer and all aspects of life. Yet this also happens with my *hitbodedut* or private prayer, because I basically say the same thing every night. I feel that I am covering everything, unless new circumstances arise. How does one prevent prayer from becoming rote or going stale? I am still trying to figure this out.

This is what I say to God every night before I go to sleep:

Please, God, keep my family on Your *derech* [path]. Keep us healthy. Keep us safe. Keep us happy. Keep us content and let all our endeavors be successful. First and foremost, I would like to thank You for the ability to speak. Then I would like to thank You for all the gifts You have given me, for all the blessings You have given me, for everything You have given me that is wonderful in this world and for everything You have given me that I must be grateful for, and there is so much. I will name the most important: my husband, my children, my speech, my family, my creative talent, my house, my food, my car, and my clothes. Then I would like to thank You for my husband, my three beautiful jewels [my children], my five grandchildren, the ability to see, hear, touch, taste, feel, breathe, speak, and express my artistic talent. I must subtract my lack of ability to walk with ease or to have proper balance.

My husband, I thank you so much for sticking it out with me, although more often than not I question your sanity. Thank you so much for taking care of all the nitty-gritty matters for our family so well. Please just stay the loved and charismatic person you are.

My eldest daughter, Orit Channah Tannenbaum Samuels, I am so proud of all the acts of *chesed* that you do and of what a beautiful woman you are, both inside and out. I am filled with pride that you are doing your *avodat kodesh* [holy work] of taking such good care of your children and bringing them up in the way of Torah, as well as everything you do to take care of me.

I am very proud of my son-in-law, Shlomo Samuels, for graduating law school, passing the bar, and practicing law. I am very grateful to him for how helpful he is to Orit, and for being such a wonderful, helpful, involved, and hands-on father. I am grateful that one can talk to him about everything and anything – real soul talks.

My second daughter, Nechama Adeena Tannenbaum Hazen, you are sweet, sensitive, caring, giving, loving, fun, funny, smart, capable, kind, and beautiful. You are very good in the kitchen, doing everything with exact precision and extreme *hashka'ah* [investment]. In your shyness, quietness, and modesty you can move mountains. You take excellent care of me. Thank You so much, Hashem, for helping Nechama figure out what she wants to do when she grows up – working with the youth. In her jobs so far both the staff and the youth love her and have great respect for her.

I am just getting to know my new son-in-law, Betzalel (Bitzi) Hazen, and so far, I am very happy with what I see. I see the adoration in his eyes for my daughter, Nechama, so I know she will be well taken care of and very happy.

When Bitzi is in the army, there must not, there cannot, there will not be a war. Bitzi must come out of the army exactly as he went in – spiritually, emotionally, mentally, and physically whole.

My son, Simcha Menachem Zev Tannenbaum, you are sweet, sensitive, caring, loving, fun, funny, smart, capable, kind, and handsome. You take excellent care of me, and we have a sharing relationship. You are a fixer, a finder, a cleaner, a doer, an organizer, a leader, and a giver par excellence.

There are two kinds of mitzvot: mitzvot between man and man, and mitzvot between man and God. The mitzvot between man and man are the most important, because in them are also included the mitzvot between man and God. Your mitzvot between man and man are exceptional. You will give someone the shirt off your back; you will give someone the pants off your legs. Not only this, but you anticipate what other people need before they even realize that they need it. And then when they finally realize that they need it, is right there waiting for them. With your leadership and giving qualities, you will do wonderful things for the nation of Israel.

I am so grateful to your rav, Rav Yonatan, for taking you under his wing and bringing you into his house. This gives you the opportunity to see a rabbi's Torah household. Hopefully these lessons will be carried into your own family when the time is right. Please may you continue to have a strong desire for and a strong love of learning Torah. May you have the *zitzfleish* [concentration] to sit and learn for an extended period of time. May you be able to leave your mark in learning just the way you leave your mark by being the person you are and by doing the things you do.

What can I say about myself, Cheri Tannenbaum? First and foremost, I'd like to thank You for giving me my speech back after forty years. There are absolutely no words to describe how grateful I am.

Thank You so much for my creative talent. When I create, I feel Your hand directing me. When I see our results I can only feel a teeny tiny bit of how You must have felt after creating Your world. My art gives me life, love, purpose, focus, joy, sanity, and a feeling of closeness to You. I am so grateful that I do not have to do laundry or scrub dishes. I do not have to wash windows. Because of my physical condition, I qualify for a full-time helper who takes care of my house. (You see, there are some perks to being ill!) I am grateful that I am free from all the domestic duties that take up 99.9 percent of a woman's time. I am grateful that I am free to create, day in and day out.

I am begging You with all my heart, my soul, and my being to help me feel, believe, and internalize that You love me more than anyone else loves me in the whole wide world.

You know my every thought.

You know my every move.

You know my every deed.

You know exactly what I need at any given time and You know exactly what is best for me, although what I think I need and what You think I need and want and what is best for me are not necessarily in sync.

Fortunately or unfortunately, You, being God, always win.

I am begging You with all my heart, my soul, and my being to help me feel, believe, and internalize that Your very essence is surrounding me, day in and day out, night in and night out, pouring down upon me Your [over-]abundance of unconditional love.

I am begging You with all my heart, my soul, and my being to help me feel, believe, and internalize that everything You do is for the good.

Every test You give me is designed specifically for me, to help me reach out of my comfort zone and actualize my spiritual, emotional, mental, and physical potential, and it is all good because You are all good. *Gam zu l'tovah* [this is also for the good]. It might not look so good to me, but this is only because I am a finite human being, and I cannot possibly fathom the Infinite Being's master plan for His world.

I am just a tiny puzzle piece in the large puzzle called the world.

I need Your help with my stinginess. The world is not all about me: I need to care for others, think of others, do for others. Thank You for letting me be financially secure thanks to the success You gave to my father for all his hard work. Everything You have given me is a gift. Gifts are meant to be shared and/or given away, so please help me to give of my resources graciously, generously, and with a smile on my face.

I also need help with my selfishness. Please help me to realize that interruptions in my well-planned day from important people and/or important things should be welcomed as an opportunity and a respite from my "in flow" creativity, rather than as something to be resented. So please help me to be able to give of my time generously, graciously, and with a smile on my face.

Please help me to connect to those important things and just get them done.

Please let all the soldiers in Israel be safe.

Please provide healing to anyone in Klal Yisrael [the community of Israel] suffering ill health.

Please let anyone in Klal Yisrael who needs a child be blessed with one.

Please let anyone in Klal Yisrael who needs a marriage partner find one.

Please let anyone in Klal Yisrael who needs help with a mental illness receive that help.

Please let anyone in Klal Yisrael who needs help with making a living get that help.

Thank you so much that all the members of my nuclear family are all healthy and thriving. Let us all continue in this way, and let us know no *tzaar* [pain, trouble].

Thank you so much that my mother is healthy and thriving. Let her continue to be so, and let her know no *tzaar*.

Thank you so much that my sisters, brothers, children, grand-children, and all their spouses are healthy and thriving. Let them continue to be so, and let them know no *tzaar*.

Thank you so much that Harvey's brothers, sisters, children, grandchildren, and their spouses are healthy and thriving. Let them continue to be so, and let them know no *tzaar*.

One last very important request: Please give me all the big, painful tests, and save the small, manageable ones for my family. I can handle it. My forty-five years of suffering have developed within me a very high pain threshold, and these muscles are constantly working on overdrive.

Thanks so much for listening to me.

Saying this in my own words gives me a feeling of connection to God. I feel listened to, purged, and much lighter after getting all of this off my chest.

I am so grateful for the opportunity to have my experiences and message be heard.

Appendix 1: Letters from Family and Friends

Before My Illness

> I am just trying to remember what kind of a person I was before this illness.

I asked people closest to me to write what they remembered about me before I became ill. I was not looking for accolades, but just trying to piece together my life, and remember what kind of a person I was before this illness.

FROM MY MOTHER

You were not a difficult child. You started to become a "terrible teen" when we moved to Vancouver. It was not a move you wanted, and you made that quite known by your behavior. In Edmonton, you used to iron your hair or put it up on frozen orange juice cans. In Vancouver, you let it go natural. You were truly the new girl on the block in Vancouver, and the guys flocked to the house.

You were very popular in school, and girls turned to you for support and to share their secrets and get your advice. Funnily enough, you abdicated the role of big sister at home and let Marc be the host if any friends came over. Marc also ran your campaign when you were nominated to be queen of the school... and you won.

A couple of times, in high school, you tried to change your grades on your report card, when you did not do well, but you did it so sloppily that it was easily detected. My disappointment in you then was that you tried to cheat, and that meant that I couldn't trust you entirely. Little did I know what else I was missing.

At some point, you became interested in yoga and worked very hard at it. You could suck your stomach in almost to your backbone and stand on your head. You actually went to some island for a workshop on yoga.

You loved sewing even then, and I bought you a small sewing machine on which you sewed some of your clothes.

You began your first year of university at the University of British Columbia, and you continued to be rebellious. You would bring friends home, and when I walked into the room, you usually didn't bother to introduce me. When I introduced myself and asked the men, especially, to stand when giving their names and shaking hands, you got very angry and said you would not bring your friends home anymore.

When Marc came home from his year in Israel and went to his first Shabbaton [youth group retreat over Shabbat] with Rabbis Marvin Hier and Pinchas "Pinky" Bak and began to explore his heritage, you were already into being a vegetarian and moving out of the house – until Dad dragged you back again.

I was disturbed about the direction you were going and asked that you give Judaism a month (the same amount of time you had spent with the yoga group) with Rabbi Hier. You finished that month looking like you had a halo over your head. You were content, sweet, smiling, and decided to go to Stern College the next year.

You and Marc went to Shabbatons in Los Angeles and Vancouver, and you met Harvey while you were living in New York. Harvey

asked you to go with him to Washington, DC, for Nixon's inauguration, and the rest is history.

My brother Harry took a picture of you wearing multiple necklaces as an ad for his jewelry store. Maybe that's where your jewelry
mania comes from.

Now in your adult life, your history is still being written. Despite
your illness, you are a wife and a mother to three wonderful children.

You have set an example of strength and spirituality that is to be
envied and is a beacon to all who have come in contact with you.

FROM MY SISTER LISA

What do I remember about you? You told me you were allergic to
me so I couldn't touch you if we were sitting near one another in
the car. You were absolutely gorgeous and wore lots of makeup. I
always tried to sneak into your room and watch you get dressed in
your jeans, big belt, and tight tops. You straightened your hair every
night and wrapped it around orange juice cans.

When we were older and got hippier, you made me and Wendy
make your carob ball things that you then sold at the health food
store – and kept the money!

You always had a boyfriend, and you always had girlfriends
around, a real posse of close-knit friends. You didn't pay me a great
deal of attention when I was younger, and then I remember you
going off to college.

I remember you coming home with Harvey for the first time and
how gorgeous you both looked together.

I remember you finding your symptoms and us thinking you
shouldn't rush to get married in case something we hadn't found
yet was really wrong with you.

I remember you going forward and going trousseau shopping
with you. And again, as always, you had great friends around to shop
with, have fun with, and celebrate the wedding together.

FROM MY FIRST COUSIN LINDA MARON

We had great fun together when we were kids. You were tall and thin (compared to me, virtually a midget), with beautiful, thick, wavy blond hair. You were very smart and when we were nine, you were a great speller.

I have memories of Palm Springs and Hawaii. And of summer in Los Angeles when you were sixteen and you worked with Shelley at my dad's office. My mother was going nuts trying to keep tabs on you. Men used to brake in their cars to look at you walking down the street because you were so beautiful and had a great figure. Really! I was jealous because I was short, flat-chested, couldn't fit into cute clothes, and looked ten years old. You and Shelley were doing fashion and makeup stuff all summer. Boohoo! I felt left out.

You became anorexic and wouldn't eat one iota of food during a Christmas vacation in Palm Springs. You didn't speak – to anyone. I was so sad because I didn't understand what was going on, and you wouldn't talk to me.

FROM MY BEST FRIEND FROM JUNIOR HIGH,
JENNY ZOTTENBERG SINGER

I remember you being obsessed with boys! You had a few crushes on guys that made you the typical dizzy dame! I remember you snuck out of your house once to see someone when you were grounded – something that was often enforced at your house. I guess you could say you were a little defiant and a bit of a risk taker! Your dad came to my house looking for you, and I knew you were in big trouble when he was out and about doing a search and rescue.

You had the most beautiful curly blond head of hair, and I recall we both spent hours with big curlers made of baby food cans when we attempted to straighten our unruly curls!

My fondest memories were of escorting you to the skating rink to put blades on for the first time. I grew up at the rink, so it was one of my favorite pastimes hanging out and feeling so free on the ice. I remember we skipped home economics class one day to buy your skates, and the first time you put them on, you gave me quite a chuckle because you looked like Bambi on ice! You were a trooper for making the effort and not worried about looking foolish!

Cher, all I know for sure is that you never had any trouble talking or expressing yourself. Things did change a few years after you moved to Vancouver. I can't really say when I noticed the difference. You went through your yoga period where you looked like a Biafran refugee. You were all big hair and skinny everywhere else. You came to visit with your packsack full of nuts and berries and stood on your head, meditated and ate little. When I came to Vancouver to visit, I remember starting to see changes each time – mostly with how you were expressing yourself. But not until your wedding did it occur to me how dramatic things had become.

FROM RABBI AVI WEISS,
MY FIRST RABBI AT STERN COLLEGE

I only have the sweetest memories going back before your illness. The most vivid were the days when you sat right in front of me as we studied Bereshit [Genesis] together at Stern. What came through for me was this deep emotional connection that you felt with Torah as you began your journey to live an observant life. Hardly a session passed that I did not see you literally cry as you studied the words of the great [biblical commentator] Rashi. Those tears coupled with a beautiful smile spoke to an inner beauty that you possess and have always had.

There is one incident that really jumps off the page. I'm not sure you remember, but after the first test, you caught me walking in front of the school and said you had to talk to me about something important. You proceeded to tell me that you were sitting too close to Joanne Rosenwald and may have seen a word on her paper. And you asked that I penalize you by lowering your grade. That was one of the greatest moments of my teaching. I think you got a 95, and when you told me that story, I turned it into 100+.

There are other great memories. One was when I was speaking at Beth Jacob many years later on the topic of when bad things happen to good people. When I was through on that Sunday morning, a striking woman came up to me, peering, looking at me. She didn't say a word and, after some long seconds, disappeared. There was something angelic about that individual. I asked a few moments later if anybody knew who this person was. And someone responded, Cheri Belzberg. I ran out of the synagogue looking for you, literally running through the streets, but couldn't find you.

Those were the days when you could hardly communicate because of the dreadful disease, but standing before me as you did, in your own way you communicated more powerfully than I have ever heard.

I pray that you are able to step back and realize what you have accomplished. You have raised a beautiful family, you are living in Efrat, and, for me and thousands of others, you are a profile in courage, a hero's hero, a gift from God. May it continue for many years to come.

FROM A FRIEND AT STERN COLLEGE,
JOANNE ROSENWALD AUMAN

So there we were in Rabbi Avi Weiss's Torah class. We both sat in the front row. Of course, Rabbi Weiss broke the ice, and I found out you were a fellow Canadian. You impressed me as natural, beautiful and friendly. I was determined to make you my friend. (Thank God, I was successful – you were a willing accomplice.) You were fun! You laughed easily, especially at my dumb jokes. (Some things don't change.) We had good times in class. When Rabbi Weiss realized that we were friends, he invited us for Shabbat several times. We were also fellow vegetarians and brownie lovers. You were different – not at all run of the mill. You had a "story," but that wasn't it. I can't put my finger on it – there was something magnetic about you. You were easy to love, easygoing, easy to talk to, smart, and spiritual.

You took meticulous but illegible notes. I now know that was part of the condition. You had great questions and a real thirst for knowledge. You and Harvey were "movie stars" in that picture of Nixon's inauguration.

I loved meeting your family. I remember we went to Papa Joe's, the Italian Moshe Peking.

You were a great kid. You were real.

I have written this in the past tense, but all these characteristics still apply. I am grateful that at a young age, I was able to pick you out and now keep you! All those years, you made sure we stayed connected. You never gave up on me. Oh, my, it's such a long time ago. But things aren't that different, are they?

You know I love you, and I cherish our friendship.

FROM A FRIEND AT STERN COLLEGE,
BONNIE NATHAN SUSSMAN

Cheri, I remember you during your college days at Stern College. You were very beautiful, waifish, soft-spoken, and eager to learn Torah. I remember the excitement when you and Harvey went to the presidential inauguration and the inaugural ball. I remember the excitement around going to your wedding as a bridesmaid. You were an amazingly beautiful bride and still are.

Letters from My Children

| They shared from their hearts.

I asked my children to write about their memories of growing up with an atypical mother. They shared from their hearts about what the experience was like for them.

FROM ORIT

Growing up with a "special" mother was not easy, yet I learned to cope, and from this I am who I am. It molded me into the person I am today.

Going back to my childhood memories, I remember that any time I would invite a new friend over to play, I would always have to prepare and tell them that my mom is different.

Telling the story made me stronger, yet I did have times when I would be embarrassed or shy. For example, walking outside with my mom while she would be sitting on her scooter chair or if she would be physically walking with me, dealing with that feeling of people staring at us, glancing back as we walked by.

It wasn't easy, but today, I walk with my mom in pride, and if people stare, I just stare back with a smile.

I walk with her in pride and no shame at all.

Today, and as I became older, I knew that not only is my mom special and different, but I am lucky to even be in this world since doctors gave her no chance when it came to having kids. My parents told me that they named me Orit because once they had me, I brought light into this world.

I thank my mom for trying and not giving up, and I thank her for bringing me into this world.

My mother is a true role model and hero.

FROM NECHAMA

My mom is just like any mom – we would play games, she'd sit next to me while I fell asleep at night, tell me to do my homework, make me food, and wait for me when I came back from school.

At first as a little girl I was a bit embarrassed of her because growing up with a mother who has a disability sometimes needed an explanation. I'd have to explain to my friends who would come for a play date that they didn't need to be scared of my mom, and that if they didn't understand her it was OK, I would let them know what she was saying.

I remember walking around the streets, holding her arm and watching all the different reactions of people when they saw her pass by. Later on when I was older, I would stare back at them.

It was a basic thing to be there by her side and support her wherever she went, explaining what she said if people didn't understand her.

Besides that, we would always make fun of the situation that she lives with a disability (in a good way, of course). Most of the time it would be a benefit for us – we would be able to cut lines in Disneyland or in the supermarket, get great parking spaces, and more. My mom would not be embarrassed to say out loud, "I have a disability."

My mom always had interesting taste in clothing. When I was a young teen and was out with her, I often felt embarrassed and would say to her, "What are you wearing?!"

But as I got older, I got over it and could say she has special taste – you can see it in her art. I even let her wear something she made to my wedding.

All parents have their rules and sayings that they tell to us as kids while we're growing up, hoping we are listening and will fulfill their wishes. So my mom had hers and never held back from saying them to us at any time. From that and more, I have learned a lot from my mom and always would be amazed at how she never gives up and keeps on doing what she is doing – living her life as she wants and not letting her condition stop her.

So growing up with a mom with a disability is all I know.

And I am thankful for that.

FROM SIMCHA

To grow up with my mother who has a disability was normal for me.

When I was available I would always be with her to go shopping on her Kalnoit, to clean the house, etc.

When I got my license, I was then able to drive her places and pick her up. My mom always told me that this isn't the way it's supposed to be – a child isn't supposed to take care of his mother. A mother is supposed to take care of her child. To this very day, she still says this and apologizes profusely.

My mother always asked me when I was at school, "Aren't you embarrassed because I have a disability?" I always said no. It doesn't bother me. It's normal for me – this is what I have.

Look at what you have and thank God for it, and don't compare to others.

Every time I was going to bring a friend home, she would always ask me her famous question, "Did you tell your friend about my condition?" My mother wanted to make sure that my friends would feel comfortable and not be scared.

Sometimes people used to ask me, "Is this your grandmother?" and I would say, "No, this is my mother."

When I went to high school, my mother would come to the PTA meetings, and I always held her arm when we walked. People were looking at the situation, but they were also looking at her outfits that she made.

People would always say to my mother, "You have such a good son who takes good care of you."

I was always my mother's translator to the world, because I grew up with her and understood her.

My mother doesn't let her condition stop her.

She just goes and does.

Appendix 11: What Is Dystonia?

The Dystonia Medical Research Foundation offers the following definition and description of dystonia.

Dystonia . . . is characterized by involuntary muscle contractions and spasms. [It] comes in many forms. Some affect only localized areas of the body (such as larynx muscles, jaw and tongue muscles, neck muscles), while others affect wider areas. Dystonia often appears as a secondary condition, a major symptom of other neurological diseases. When it is unrelated to another disease, dystonia generally does not impact cognition or intelligence or shorten one's life span. Although the causes of the disease are not yet known, the localized (or focal) form presents disproportionately in individuals who perform high-precision hand movements, like musicians, engineers, artists and architects. This seems to indicate that environmental factors may play a role.

Dystonia is a movement disorder characterized by involuntary muscle contractions that cause abnormal movements and or postures. The movements can be repetitive and twisting. There may be an associated jerky tremor which is typically present with specific positions. Dystonia is often activated or worsened by voluntary movements, and symptoms may "overflow" into nearby muscles. Dystonia is sometimes painful, often depending on the area of the body affected.

Dystonia presents in many forms, involving various body areas and multiple causes. Experts believe dystonia is the result of excessive signals arising from the brain that cause target muscles to contract inappropriately. However, the exact reason why the brain delivers these excessive signals is not completely understood.

Dystonia is the third most common movement disorder after essential tremor and Parkinson's disease. The exact incidence and prevalence of dystonia are not known, but studies suggest no fewer than three hundred thousand people are affected in the U.S. and Canada. Dystonia affects men women and children of all ages and backgrounds.

Age of Onset

Dystonia can occur at any age from infancy to adulthood. Some forms of dystonia are specific to certain age groups. Dystonia that begins in childhood is more likely to have an identifiable cause – for example, a gene mutation or specific disease/condition known to cause dystonia – and is more likely to progress from one area of the body to other muscle groups. Dystonia that begins in adulthood is less likely to progress extensively.

How Does Dystonia Affect the Body?

The areas of the body typically targeted by dystonia are the neck, face, jaw, lids and brow, hands, feet, limbs or vocal cords. It is possible for dystonia to begin on one area of the body and spread to involve additional muscle groups. Symptoms may remain fairly consistent throughout the day or fluctuate often in recognizable patterns related to sleep and waking.

When dystonia affects a single body area it is called focal dystonia.

Segmental dystonia affects two or more connected body areas. Multifocal dystonia affects two or more areas of the body that are not connected. Generalized dystonia refers to dystonia that affects the limbs, torso and other major body areas simultaneously. When dystonia affects muscles on one side of the body, it is called hemidystonia.

Dystonia that only occurs when a person does a specific activity – for example, a musician who develops symptoms only when playing an instrument – is described as task-specific.

Movement symptoms that occur only in episodes may be referred to as paroxysmal dyskinesia.

How Is Dystonia Treated?

Because each person with dystonia is unique, treatment must be highly customized to the needs of the individual. Doctors may recommend a combination of approaches: oral medications, botulinum neurotoxin injections, physical therapy or other supportive therapies and surgical procedures. Complementary techniques such as relaxation and stress reduction practices may also be beneficial. The type of doctor who is typically trained to diagnose and treat dystonia is a neurologist with special training in movement disorders, often called a movement disorder specialist. Otolaryngologists, neuro-ophthalmologists, ophthalmologists and other health care providers may also treat dystonias that fall within their practices.

Is Dystonia Fatal?

Dystonia is almost never fatal. In rare cases, a person with a severe generalized dystonia may experience secondary effects that require prompt or emergency medical attention. Such circumstances are treatable and most people recover fully. Dystonia may occur as a symptom of multiple degenerative diseases and these conditions may affect life span.

What Can I Expect?

The dystonia experience can vary from person to person, depending on the diagnosis and nature of the symptoms. While some cases are relatively mild, others may progress in severity. In most cases, dystonia does require ongoing medical management. In addition to the dystonic symptoms, many individuals experience fatigue and or pain that affect daily activities. Tension and anxiety do not cause dystonia, but symptoms may worsen during periods of emotional or mental stress. Because therapies must be tailored to the individual patient, it can take time to find the right treatment plan that is most beneficial. Research suggests that individuals with dystonia may be at increased risk for depression and anxiety, so caring for one's emotional and mental health may be an important part of the overall treatment plan.

How Is Dystonia Diagnosed?

At this time, there is no single medical test to confirm the diagnosis of dystonia. The diagnosis rests on the ability of a qualified doctor to recognize the symptoms and rule out other possibilities. Genetic testing is available to identify specific mutations known to cause dystonia, for example, TOR1A/DYT12, ThAP1/DYT6, ATP1A3/DYT12. A neurologist with special training in movement disorders is typically the sub-specialist referral made to diagnose and treat dystonia.

How Is Dystonia Classified?

There are many forms of dystonia and the outward symptoms may appear quite different. Dystonia is classified according to the clinical signs and the cause. Doctors look at these factors to guide diagnosis and treatment. Clinical signs include the age at which symptoms began, how symptoms are distributed on the body, any special characteristics of the symptoms (for example, are symptoms persistent or do they only occur while doing a specific task), and associated features such as additional movement disorders or neurological symptoms.

In many cases of dystonia, the cause is not known. In other cases, the onset of dystonia can be attributed to a specific cause or trigger. These may include genetic mutations, brain injury, exposure to certain medications, or additional neurological or metabolic disorders.

Professional musicians may be at risk of dystonia related to performing an instrument. In very rare cases, dystonia can be attributed to a combination of neurological and psychological causes.

The Dystonia Medical Research Foundation is a 501c3 non-profit organization that has served the dystonia community since 1976. The DMRF funds medical research toward improved treatments and a cure, promotes awareness and education, and provides support resources for affected individuals and families.

For more information, contact dystonia@dystonia-foundation.org

Appendix III: Inspirational Quotes

When we see people with disabilities from our limited perspectives, we have separated ourselves from them. When we treat people with disabilities . . . effortlessly and without judgment – that is when we, too, can see the spirit of each individual human.

> Rachel Sokol, "No Barriers or Awkwardness," https:// www.chabad.org/library/article_cdo/aid/3236794 /jewish/No-Barriers-or-Awkwardness.htm; used by permission of Chabad.org

We don't understand the purpose for all of our difficult sojourns, persecutions, troubles or ailments. But throughout them all, G-d assures us that He is with us. We are not alone; G-d hears and He cares. That may not take away our pain, or our suffering, but it is comforting to know that G-d is by our side.

In those heart-wrenching moments, when we feel like we cannot continue, G-d is holding our hands, holding us up and helping us to take one step after another.

> Chana Weisberg, "You Are Never Alone," December 17, 2017, https://www.chabad.org/blogs/blog_cdo/aid /3865115/jewish/You-Are-Never-Alone.htm; used by permission of Chabad.org

All of these struggles, all of the complications and obstacles of life, are sent to us as an opportunity for to spur us along towards [the] greatness of the creation of a mind. These small struggles are all intended as goads to prod us towards the realization that we must turn to Hashem. Every small challenge that you face is actually challenging you to recognize that Hashem is everything, and that He's your address for anything you want.

> Rabbi Wohlhendler, "Parshas Eikev – Becoming a Man of Prayer," *Toras Avigdor: Rav Avigdor Miller on the Parsha; Adapted from His Tapes, Sforim and Writings of Talmidim,* https://torasavigdor.org/parshas-eikev-becoming-a-man -of-prayer-2/; used by permission of Toras Avigdor

Rabbi Akiva's statement, "Everything that G-d does is for the good," implies that since the situation is ordained by Divine Providence, G-d is behind it. Therefore, we can be sure that it will eventually lead to a favorable outcome.

In other words, the situation itself may be painful or unpleasant, but it will lead to a positive outcome. If we were to know the positive results from the outset, we would decide that it is worth enduring this negative experience for the sake of the positive experience. Rabbi Akiva taught that even when a person does not have such foreknowledge, he should have the faith that G-d is controlling his experience and should therefore accept everything with happiness.

> Shloma Majeski, "Being Happy at All Times," *The Chassidic Approach to Joy,* https://www.chabad.org /library/article_cdo/aid/88577/jewish/Chapter-2-Being -Happy-At-All-times.htm; used by permission of Chabad. org

When we are confronted with a challenge, we should view it as an opportunity for spiritual growth rather than try to avoid it. Comfort and contentment can cause us to lose sight of priorities, weakening our sense of urgency in our Divine mission. Physical or spiritual adversity can shock us out of this indifference, under-mining our self-assurance and affording us the opportunity to advance in our relationship with G-d by breaking through the obstacle.

> *Daily Wisdom: Inspiring insights on the Torah portion from the Lubavitcher Rebbe*, translated and adapted by Moshe Wisnefsky, https://www.chabad.org/dailystudy /dailywisdom_cdo/aid/2944942/jewish/Monday -Embracing-Spiritual-Challenges.htm; used by permission of Chabad.org

There is no "I can't." God can make anything possible in our lives. We need to wake up every day and look at the road ahead, saying: With God's help, I can do this. There is a pain threshold we think we can't get past, a level of discomfort we think we can't bear. But when we push past it, we often realize that limit was really just a false line we drew in our own minds.

> Sara Debbie Gutfreund, "Lessons from Running," Aish. com, January 16, 2016, https://www.aish.com/sp/pg /Lessons-from-Running.html; used by permission of Aish. com

Every time a person faces a challenge he can create a great *kiddush Hashem* [sanctification of God's name] by recognizing that God has not abandoned him, that God is closer to him more than ever before and knows precisely what he is doing. When we know that God is with us we receive a great deal of encouragement and the ability to overcome any challenge that comes our way.

> Orit Esther Riter, dailydoseofemuna.com; used by permission of Orit Esther Riter

It's all from God.
>   God is my father.
>   It must be good.
>   The ultimate best for me.

What is the message God is sending me?

Orit Esther Riter, dailydoseofemuna.com; used by permission of Orit Esther Riter

God has more information than we do; thus we cannot judge Him and say He is doing something bad. We trust God and say, "I haven't yet figured out why, but God knows this is for the best."

"Suffering: Why?" https://www.aish.com/atr/Suffering _Why.html; used by permission of Aish.com

In the morning prayers, we thank God for giving the rooster the intuition and ability to differentiate between day and night. Rabbi Nachman of Breslov says that we also have the ability to differentiate. When does the rooster differentiate? When does it sense day? When it senses light coming at the darkest moment of the night. The last part of the night is the darkest moment of the night. Even when things seem so very dark, the rooster has the ability to sense and understand that it will be light. No matter how dark our life may seem, no matter how difficult it may seem, we need to say, "Thank you, Hashem, for giving me the ability to sense that even in my darkest moment, light will come."

Rabbi Yechiel Spero, *Inspiration Daily*, Yeshiva Ateres Shimon; used by permission of Rabbi Yechiel Spero

When people refer to negative occurrences in life as punishments, they operate along materialistic guidelines. According to this view, the "bad" thing is anything which stands in the way of a person's experiencing the pleasures and comforts of life. Losing a job means that there will be less money to get things one wants to have, to do the things one wants to do. An illness spells pain. There is frustration with not being able to enjoy sports, or even to do simple chores at one's will. There seems to be no answer as to why bad things happen – natural calamities, wars, death. One draws the conclusion that it must be that G-d is a cruel G-d, quick to punishment. This view fills one with anxiety and dread of the future. If it is good now, it means that it will get bad at some point.

The spiritual approach offers another explanation to life's seemingly painful events. The underlying principle of creation is that G-d made this world for the purpose of serving Him with complete devotion and self-abandonment, making this material existence into a dwelling place for Him. He is the Creator, and He causes everything to run according to His will. With every thing that happens to us, whether good or bad, we can learn how to serve Him a little better, how to draw down His presence a little closer. The challenges set in front of us are never greater than what we can handle. G-d is not only behind us, encouraging and cheering as we muster the strength to keep going, but He is beside us, breathing energy into us, and carrying us in His arms when we are unable to walk by ourselves. He is not out to break us, but to make us.

Losing a job, becoming ill or any other calamity one can think of are not punishments. At first, they cause us to reach deeper and deeper into our own resources, until we realize that we can't do it without Him. From that, the realization that *nothing* is possible without Him begins to infiltrate our minds and hearts, changing our frame of reference on the world from self-centered to G-d-centered, exactly as He wants it to be. I cannot perceive a source of greater comfort and security.

> Gittle Gesina, "Punishments or Gifts?" https://www
> .chabad.org/library/article_cdo/aid/132656/jewish
> /Punishments-or-Gifts.htm; used by permission of
> Chabad.org

Who isn't suffering nowadays? We're surrounded by tragedy, difficulty and challenges. . . . Yet, can the source of some of our misery possibly be that we view our lives in a limited way, believing that what we hold now represents how we always were and will be?

The truth is, of course, that our world is just a tiny snapshot of the infinite cosmic worlds, and we are seeing but a tiny dot of the full picture. But moreover, even within the here and now of our physical world, everything remains in a state of flux. We may not be aware of it, but at every moment there is enormous change. The shift may occur so slightly as to be imperceptible to our eyes and minds, but it is taking place....

Perhaps God's message...to us in our moments of misery [is that] we can connect to divinity with "I will be what I will be" – the power to be....

When the blackness seems overpowering, when the tedious monotony is driving us to the brink of insanity, we can take comfort in the realization that nothing in our world remains static.

Not our present challenges. Nor who we are.

You, your life and your circumstances are an integral part of G-d's cosmic plan, emerging anew every instance. The present is only what we have brought from our pasts, and what we will use to forge our immediate futures.

There is no static "is." There is only what we were – and most importantly, what we choose to become.

> Chana Weisberg, "A Message of Hope," December 27, 2015, https://www.chabad.org/blogs/blog_cdo/aid/3171054 /jewish/A-Message-of-Hope.htm; used by permission of Chabad.org

When it appears to us that something is wrong in the way G-d runs the world, G-d wants us to question Him. But at the same time, we must continue to believe absolutely in G-d's reality and goodness.

> *Daily Wisdom: Inspiring insights on the Torah portion from the Lubavitcher Rebbe,* translated and adapted by Moshe Wisnefsky, https://www.chabad.org/dailystudy /dailywisdom_cdo/aid/2944716/jewish/Sunday-Seeing -G-d.htm; used by permission of Chabad.org

It is always important to remember that when we go through our own tests, *"shnayim mikrah v'echad targum"* [read the original biblical passage twice, and then once in translation]. God's dictation of the way He assumes and conducts the world, is twice, but the *echad*, the one, is the translation of it. There will be things we don't understand. There will be times when Hashem acts in a manner where the *targum*, the translation and understanding are missing; why are we going through this if we don't understand it? Nevertheless, there will be a *geula* (redemption) from that *mitzrayim* (exile in Egypt). There will be a time when we understand everything.

> Rabbi Yechiel Spero, *Inspiration Daily*, Yeshiva Ateres Shimon; used by permission of Rabbi Yechiel Spero

Our relationship to Hashem is often dependent on His ability to fulfill our needs and desires. As human beings, we naturally desire pleasure and comfort. When we are showered with what we define as good, we generally do not question Hashem's ways. If life events do not clash with our perception of good or comfortable, then we are not provoked to question His divine plan. We merely take things for granted and expect them to flow as we believe they should. However, if our needs and comforts are not met, we may begin to question His ways. This mistaken outlook is a product of our limited egos, a lack of knowledge of the full picture and a lack of emunah that everything that happens is for the best.

> Orit Esther Riter, dailydoseofemuna.com; used by permission of Orit Esther Riter

As long as we are accepting and not asking, "Why me?" we can feel pain and utilize it for our benefit with a full heart.

> Rabbi Abraham J. Twerski; used by permission of Rabbi Abraham J. Twerski

Although it may seem counterintuitive, the moment of our greatest pain and sorrow is the moment when we can feel Hashem's embrace. At a time of *hester panim* [God's hiddenness], Hashem is very close. Sadly, all too often, when we are struck by troubles and misfortunes, we close our hearts. We shut our lips from prayer and turn away from Hashem. We can instead offer up our pain to Hashem and in doing so, access His love. These are times that are supercharged; from within them, we can gain a relationship with our Maker that is laden with love.

> Rebbetzin Shira Smiles, "Eshet Lot: Salt of the Earth";
> used by permission of Rebbetzin Shira Smiles

Cruel comments are made by the ignorant and by those who cannot see past the obvious to find the grandeur in other people.

> John J. Heney, *The Thunder Within: A True Story* (Renfrew,
> Ontario: General Store Publishing House, 2002); used by
> permission of John J. Heney

We triumph when we are spiritually strong. Victory begins where ego ends. When we are fighting a personal battle, we need to recognize that the impossible is possible as long as we acknowledge that all results come from the Divine will. Hashem controls everything. Anything is possible as long as we take the first step for Hashem's sake. We stand a great chance of meriting *siyatta d'shmaya* [godly assistance] if we undertake a genuine act of *mesirut nefesh* [self-sacrifice] – an act which seems too difficult or defies human logic. In order to receive this Divine assistance, we must take that first step outside our comfort zone. If we have invested normal measures of *hishtadlut* [effort], but the way is still blocked and there still appears to be no relief, we must try to completely give ourselves over to *ratzon* [the will of] Hashem. Practically speaking, this may include letting go of our worries and uplifting our *bitachon* [trust] and increasing our connection to Hashem by growing in another area of Yiddishkeit, or continuing to live life as though the situation has already materialized. Time and again, when a person finds himself being tested to go outside his natural habitat, he is given superpowers that he knows are not his or humanly possible. So too, when we let go and let in God, we receive strength to cope, hope and survive under the most difficult circumstances. Hashem is waiting to pour down miracles for those who have emunah to surrender their *nefesh* [soul]. Know that there is no one to rely on but Hashem.

> Orit Esther Riter, dailydoseofemuna.com; used by permission of Orit Esther Riter

We need to know that Hashem is closest to us during our most difficult moments. He comes at times of hardship and pain to be with us to encourage us and to tell us, "I wish it could be different now but this is what you need. Do not worry, I am here to help you." Whenever we are in pain, God is also in pain.

> Orit Esther Riter, dailydoseofemuna.com; used by permission of Orit Esther Riter

Everything Hashem does come from His love for us. When God tests us, there are three negative conclusions that come to us:

1. Hashem isn't fair, and I am being punished for no reason.
2. I am bad, so I am being punished.
3. The world is crazy, and I am in terrible danger.

To get out of this mindset and into a Torah mindset, we need to think and realize that God loves us and is giving us these tests so we should know our greatness. We know our greatness when we are stressed and act in a Torah way.

Our spiritual powers are our *middot* [character traits].

God wants us to not be so attached to this world, because when we have it so good, we don't need Him.

Don't focus on what you don't have; focus on what you do have.

> Dr. Miriam Adahan; used by permission of Dr. Miriam Adahan

When we get hurt or afflicted, it is not a punishment out of vengeance.... It is a correction out of love. If we would know why Hashem was doing it and the benefit we receive as a result, we would ask for it ourselves.

"Hashem's Infinite Love," http://www.divreichizuk.com /id74.html; used by permission

One of the most difficult parts of any hardship is feeling that we are going through it alone. We often think that nobody understands what we are experiencing. However, there is a remedy. We would have so much comfort if we internalized the fact that we are never alone. Hashem knows exactly what we are experiencing. He knows how hard it is, and he feels it even more than we do.

"We Are Not Alone," Daily Emunah, https://www.ou.org /torah/machshava/daily-emunah/daily-emunah-not -alone/; used by permission

When a person faces a problem, the natural reaction might be to look at others who don't have that problem and think "why me"? Why did I have to be stuck with this? We have to understand. God gives every single person his own job to do. Everyone has his own set of challenges and tests. God gives everyone exactly what they need to achieve their purpose in the world. It doesn't matter what anybody else has. Life is about doing the best we can in the situation that God puts us in. It is so important to remember that we have no control over the results. All that matters is our effort. Everybody has a different job. We are here only to do our job. Sometimes we wish things could be different, but that is only because we can't see the bigger picture. One day it will all be explained. We will understand why we had to have each hardship. We will see how elevated we became by being strong, doing the best we can and having *emunah* that every last detail of our lives was carefully planned for us by God.

Every time we feel like saying, "I can't do this anymore," but instead, we strengthen ourselves and continue to persevere, it is so precious. The reward is unfathomable. God is righteous. He doesn't make mistakes. God knows exactly what He is doing. By accepting His will and being happy with the role that He wants us to play, we give God the greatest gift of all – our will.

> "Why Me?" Daily Emunah, https://www.ou.org/torah /machshava/daily-emunah/daily-emunah-why-me/; used by permission

Man needs God – and God wants man. Man becomes truly powerful only when he comprehends his human powerlessness. Prayer is the link between the creator and his creations. Without prayer man thinks he is God – and that unwarranted sense of ego ensures his defeat and destruction.

And that is the meaning of faith. Faith is not knowing what the future holds. It is knowing who holds the future.

Prayer defines us. Prayer gives us hope. Prayer puts into words the values we hold most precious, the people we most treasure, the ideals for which we live and for which we are prepared to give up our lives.

> Rabbi Benjamin Blech, "The San Bernardino Massacre and Prayer," December 8, 2015, https://www.aish.com /sp/pr/The-San-Bernardino-Massacre-And-Prayer.html; used by permission of Aish.com

Tefillah [prayer] is not something that you do as a *mitzvah* one time or ten times. *Tefillah is a way of life!* Tefillah means a state of existence, a frame of mind of being always in contact with Hakadosh Baruch Hu [God].

> Rabbi Wohlhendler, "Parshas Eikev – Becoming a Man of Prayer," *Toras Avigdor: Rav Avigdor Miller on the Parsha; Adapted from His Tapes, Sforim and Writings of Talmidim,* https://torasavigdor.org/parshas-eikev-becoming-a-man -of-prayer-2/; used by permission of Toras Avigdor

Davening [praying] is the struggle to make the words meaningful in our hearts. We have to work on it very hard because often we don't know what we are saying, or the translation. You have to make a *kinyon* [acquisition] on the words. The words have to mean something to you. Within the words of the *tefillah* [prayer] is the potential for you to put in anything that you're feeling. In order to do this, you have to understand the words. It's a process of taking phrases that are going to be meaningful to you. This is a challenge, an *avodah* [work] because it's not going to happen by itself. You have to punctuate your prayer with phrases that will be meaningful to you. This is done by learning the commentaries on the Torah.

There are three aspects to prayer:

1. Praise
2. Thanks
3. Asking for what you need.

Of these three, asking is the easiest. When I need something, I just ask for it. What am I asking for? I have so much, yet I don't know you, God, and I really want to. I feel the *averot* [sins] I have done are hiding you from me. I am going to change the world and make a difference. This is what you should be asking for.

People are also good at saying thank you. People who have everything won't enjoy it until they lose it. The challenge is to appreciate what we have while we have it. You will enjoy life more if you realize how much you have.

We aren't so good with praise because it makes us feel uncomfortable.

God needs me to praise him? What can we say to the infinite one? We can't grasp infinity. *Bishvili nivra ha'olam* [because of me the world was created]. I am going to change things through my prayer. We can't control things. The only thing we have is the *koach* [strength] of our prayer. God wants us to pray, to pray to him.

Rabbi Dovid Orlofsky